Blood Pressure Control

Volume 1

THOMAS G. COLEMAN
School of Medicine
Department of Physiology and Biophysics
The University of Mississippi Medical Center
Jackson, Mississippi 39216

Eden Press
MEDICAL & SCIENTIFIC PUBLISHERS

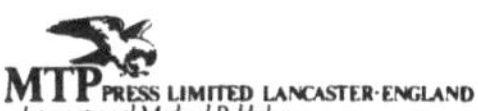
MTP PRESS LIMITED LANCASTER·ENGLAND
International Medical Publishers

ISBN 978-94-015-1330-2 ISBN 978-94-015-1328-9 (eBook)
DOI 10.1007/978-94-015-1328-9

Softcover reprint of the hardcover 1st edition 1980

Published simultaneously in Canada by
Eden Press Inc., Suite 10, 245 Victoria Avenue, Westmount, Quebec H3Z 2M6.

in the United States of America by
Eden Medical Research Inc., PO Box 51, St. Albans, VT 05478.

and in the United Kingdom and Europe by
MTP Press Limited, Falcon House, Cable Street, Lancaster, England.
(ISBN 978-94-015-1330-2)

FOREWORD

The way in which blood pressure is controlled is not well understood. I offer as evidence the spirited debates among scientists that have occurred in the past and that will probably continue for some time to come. Consider also that hypertension is a disease of significant morbidity and mortality, yet in the majority of instances the cause of the pressure elevation is unknown. And further, the wide variety of antihypertensive drugs currently used, often without a full understanding of the mechanisms involved, suggests that we often know as little about what decreases blood pressure with antihypertensive therapy as we know about what increases pressure in the first place.

This ignorance has fostered and probably justified extensive inquiries into outstanding problems of blood pressure control. The pace has quickened in the last one or two decades, and published reports germaine to the subject appear to be accumulating at an exponential rate. Hence, speaking for myself, the reviewer is faced with too little understanding and too much information.

It is clear that the control of blood pressure is complicated but it is not clear that it must remain a mystery. Certain general notions are emerging from the wealth of data now available for analysis. To name several : the kidneys appear to have a very important role or roles in blood pressure control; the level of intake of sodium chloride can have important long-term influences on blood pressure; and, the renin-angiotensin system has a much greater diversity of influences on blood pressure than previously appreciated. In this review I have tried to consolidate and generalize when it seemed appropriate at the risk of oversimplifying and/or allowing biases to foster impartiality. The reader is forewarned.

All reviews must have limits placed on the range and detail of the material covered. Consequently, many important topics have been mentioned only briefly or not at all in the pages that follow. This means that even though an extensive bibliography follows, many significant publications have not been cited. A second and much less appealing reason for an uneven review can be traced directly to the author's fallibility in ferreting out all of the new and relevant publications; for this latter deficiency, I apologize now to the scientists who have been slighted.

Several acknowledgements are in order. First, my appreciation goes to Mrs. Veda Morgan, Ms. Mary Matthes, Milton H. Davis, Jr. and a sometimes friendly local computer for assistance in preparing this photo-ready copy. Sincere thanks also go jointly to Professor Arthur C. Guyton of the University of Mississippi Medical Center, to Professor J. M. Ledingham of the London Hospital Medical College, and to many of my colleagues for sharing their enthusiasm and insight in matters of blood pressure control. Finally, I thank my wife and children for encouragement with tolerance in those many undertakings which somehow require an inexorable amount of time -- in this case, it was the preparation of the text that follows.

Thomas G. Coleman
October, 1980

CONTENTS

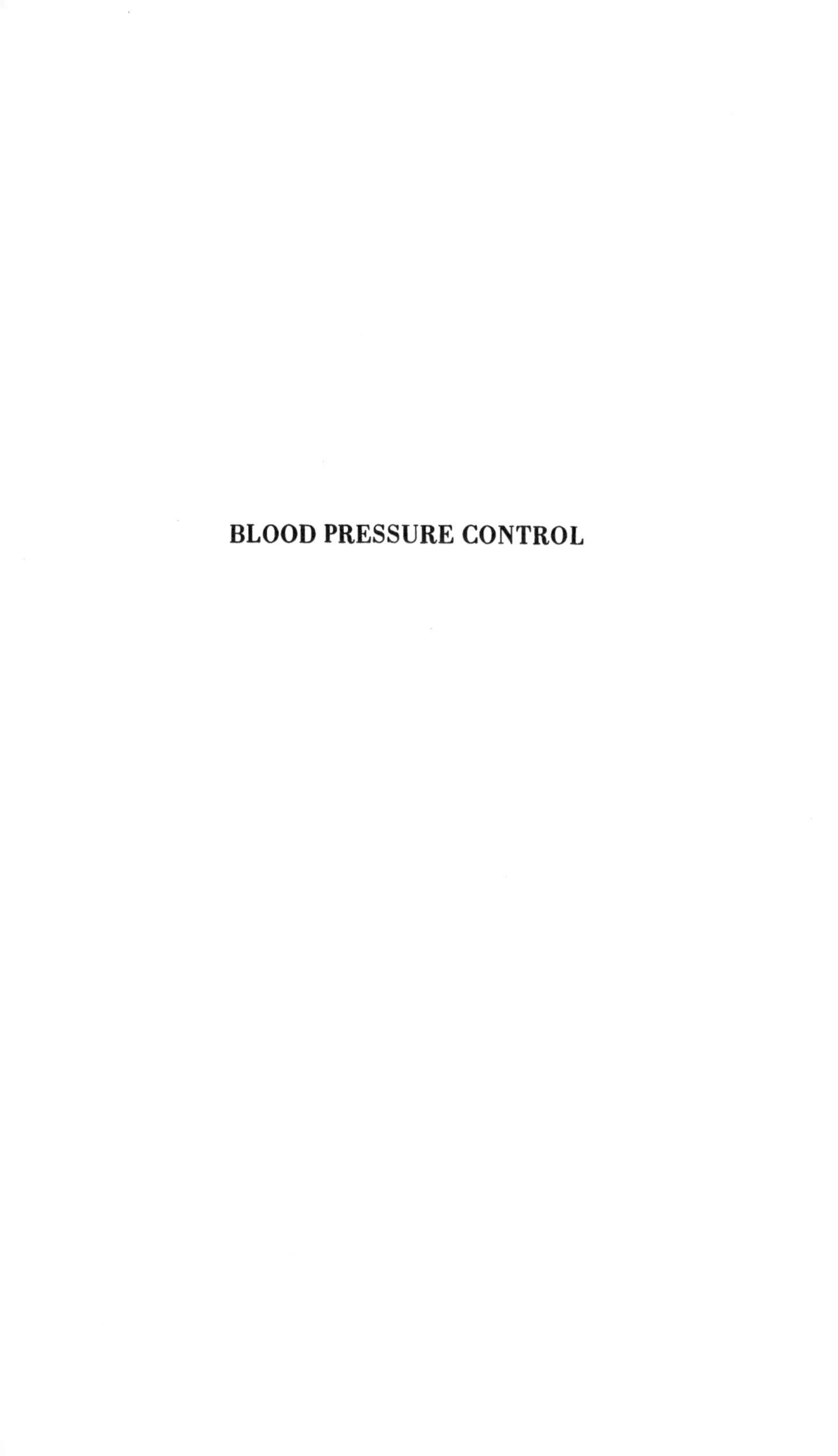

BLOOD PRESSURE CONTROL

CHAPTER 1

ARTERIAL BLOOD PRESSURE

> "In December I caused a mare to be tied down alive on her back; she was fourteen hands high, and about fourteen years of age; had a fistula of her withers, was neither very lean nor yet lusty; having laid open the left crural artery about three inches from her belly, I inserted into it a brass pipe whose bore was one sixth of an inch in diameter... I fixed a glass tube of nearly the same diameter which was nine feet in length : then untying the ligature of the artery, the blood rose in the tube 8 feet 3 inches perpendicular above the level of the left ventricle..."

This passage is from _Statical Essays : Containing Haemostaticks_, a treatise written in 1733 by an English clergyman named Stephen Hales. Although there undoubtedly was interest in arterial blood pressure before the 18th century, this experiment of sorts by the Reverend Hales is often cited (97),(346) as an early and dramatic demonstration that the blood in the arteries is under considerable pressure -- enough to elevate a column of water some five feet or more.

THE CONSTANCY OF BLOOD PRESSURE

An arterial pressure that is excessively high over an extended period causes many changes within the circulatory system leading to vascular damage and increased morbidity and mortality. Organ failure is especially apparent in the brain, heart, and kidneys. On the other hand, an arterial pressure that is too low leads most notably to insufficient perfusion of the brain, disorientation, and loss of consciousness. Normally, blood pressure resides over the long-term in a narrow band between these two extremes.

Observed values of arterial pressure are remarkably constant not only among individuals within a species but also among different mammalian species. Normal blood pressure in man is little different than normal blood pressure in horses, cows, dogs, cats, rats, and mice as an inspection of the tabulated data in (14) or (346)(Chapter 5) will show.

The giraffe is an exception (747),(952). Arterial pressures of up to 300 mm Hg at the level of the heart have been reported in this animal. It may be argued that a high arterial pressure at the origin of the aorta is required to overcome the considerable hydrostatic gradient in the giraffe's neck if proper cerebral perfusion is to be maintained when the animal is grazing in a fully upright position.

With the exception of the giraffe, and the observation that blood pressure in the rabbit is usually on the low side, arterial pressure in general is remarkably constant in mammals. If a single number was picked to characterize the mean pressure of these species in total it should probably be in the neighborhood of 100 mm Hg or 13.3 kPa.

THE CONTROL OF ARTERIAL PRESSURE

Cardiac ouput increase rapidly with the size of the animal (as expected), but it also decreases rapidly with size on a per-unit-weight basis (394). Heart rate is highly variable and ranges from about 20 beats/min in whales and elephants to about 1000 beats/min in the shrew. Blood pressure is much more constant and it has been demonstrated, at least in part, that powerful control mechanisms are responsible. In the review that follows, these mechanisms will be dissected into short-term controllers and long-term controllers. There must be overlap, of course, but this division can serve as a starting point.

Short-term control certainly involves the nervous system. The nearly immediate reflex responses to changes in posture and the neural support of arterial pressure during exercise are examples. Recently, the diversity of afferent reflex pathways coming from both the high pressure and low pressure regions of the cardiovascular system has come under intensive study. The complete importance of this very complex system or combination of systems has not yet been fully evaluated or appreciated.

Unfortunately, a detailed review of short-term control could not be incorporated into this review.

Long-term control of arterial pressure is assumed to be responsible for maintaining blood pressure from week to week and longer. A variety of processes have been implicated in long-term control : the nervous system, the renin-angiotensin system, other circulating vasoconstrictor hormones, dietary salt intake and the kidney's excretroy capacity, adrenal steroids, and others. All are plausable components of a long-term control scheme, but it has been very difficult to isolate individual contributions. Contributions may vary with time and other particulars, and they may have disparate quantitative ratings of importance. An evaluation of these individual elements of pressure control is the main thrust of blood pressure research today.

Hypertension can be considered to be a demonstation of dysfunction in the long-term blood pressure control system. Therefore, a currently very popular investigative strategy is to induce hypertension in experimental animals or to observe hypertensive patients in the clinic. Then, inferences are drawn about which components of pressure control may have caused the hypertension to occur. It is also sometimes possible to implicate components that opposed the pressure change and those that played no role at all. These considerations will resurface in the chapters that follow.

In a nutshell, those doing research in blood pressure control today are faced with the following question : What factors or factors

1. normally maintain blood pressure in humans and other mammals within a narrow range,
2. while permitting pressure in the giraffe to go to a high but appartently beneficial level,
3. while also allowing pressure to drift upward in many humans with an undesirable outcome and without any obvious cause ?

As an aside, it should be noted that Item 2. in the above list has received little (no) attention to date.

CHAPTER 2

BLOOD PRESSURE MEASUREMENT

An appreciation in the 18th century that blood in the arterial system is under considerable pressure was cited at the beginning of the previous chapter. In the subsequent two centuries techniques emerged for both the direct and indirect measurement of arterial blood pressure. Today, there is a continuing appraisal of these methods since indirect methods are vulnerable to error while the direct techniques require invasive procedures. The question of exactly what values for pressure should be considered abnormal has not yet been settled. Use of "mmHg" and "cm H2O" as standard units of pressure is slowly being replaced by the more scientific "Pascal."

A BRIEF HISTORY OF BLOOD PRESSURE MEASUREMENT

Measurement of blood pressure is now a commonplace diagnostic tool. Several historical accounts of the evolution of pressure measuring techniques are available (967), (346) but probably the best account is provided by Booth (97). Realistically, the overall development of pressure measuring techniques was the result of diverse contributions by a great many individuals; however, in retrospect several individuals and events stand out.

Stephen Hales (born 1677 - died 1761) studied biology at Cambridge and his measurement of arterial pressure in the horse in 1733 in all likelihood followed directly from an interest in the movement of sap in plants.

Jean Leonard Marie Poiseuille (born 1799 - died 1869) was a French physician and physicist who is best known for his description of the viscous and geometric components of the vascular resistance to blood flow (Poiseuille's Law). But, as a medical student in Paris in the 1820's, he devised the mercury manometer and fully demonstrated its utility.

Karl Friedrich Wilhelm Ludwig (born 1816 - died 1895) was a renown German teacher and physiologist who along with

Bowman advanced early ideas on the formation of urine by glomerular filtration. He was also an inventor who devised the kymograph for making (relatively) permanent recordings of arterial pressure and other physiological data. His idea was to add a float to a mercury manometer and to use this to create a tracing on a rotating drum. The kymograph remained the standard laboratory instrument in blood pressure research until the relatively recent development of electronic recorders.

Some alternative to direct measurement of intravascular pressure was obviously needed for human investigations. During the last half of the 19th century several indirect methods were explored. The most successful was that of Samuel Siegfried Karl Ritter von Basch (born 1837 - died 1905). His device developed an external counterpressure over an artery and the pressure needed to just produce vascular collapse was noted and recorded. Von Basch's device was widely used but the measurement errors that attend such an approach rendered it less than perfect.

Then in 1896, Scipione Riva-Rocci (born 1863 - died 1936) an Italian physician invented a pneumatic cuff that encircled the arm; it remains basically unchanged today. The cuff was progressively deflated until pulsations could be pulpated and the (systolic) pressure was noted. Diastolic pressure could not be measured.

In 1905, N. C. Korotkoff (born 1874 - died 1920) a Russian surgeon described the auscultatory method. A stethoscope was used to detect sounds distal to a Riva-Rocci pressure cuff that could characteristically be associated with both systolic and diastolic pressure. This method was slowly accepted as a superior way to measure blood pressure in humans.

There have been two additional significant events in recent years. One was the development of the modern electronic recorder or polygraph. The other was the development of compact pressure transducers which offer sensitivity and frequency response that are superior to the mercury manometer.

ACCURACY OF PRESSURE MEASUREMENTS

Two problems must be addressed when accuracy is being considered. One is whether or not a particular method of pressure measurement will give an accurate value for pressure at the moment the data is being collected; this concern applies only to indirect methods of course. The second problem is whether or not the recorded value can be considered to be representative of pressure over a longer timespan -- for instance, over 24 hours for once-a-day measurements.

Measurements in humans

The vast majority of determinations have been indirect, using the auscultatory form of sphygmomanometry. A pressure cuff is used to meter blood flow and a stethoscope is used to listen for the sounds that characterize systolic and diastolic pressure. Pressures by this method have been compared to values taken directly from indwelling cannulae (776), (891), (994) and sphygmomanometry has been found to be relatively accurate if care is taken to use the proper pressure cuff size (30).

Even though pressure can be accurately measured by sphygmomanometry, the values obtained may not be representative of true, average arterial pressure. A single determination in an individual is likely to overestimate blood pressure. Presumably this is caused by the more frightening aspects of a trip to the doctor and by underlying worries about debilitating disease. The subject's familiarity with the procedures involved and with the environment is probably important, since values for pressure usually decrease with repeated measurements (761). Pressures recorded at home are often lower than those recorded in the clinic (39).

Direct intra-arterial recording has recently been used to continuously monitor arterial pressure in ambulatory subjects (72), (73), (594). A definite circadian rhythm has been observed, with the lowest pressures occuring during sleep, around 3 AM, and much higher pressures occuring during the daytime (73). A recent monograph describes the current activity in this area (157).

Its quite likely, then, that the true 24-hour mean arterial pressure is considerably less than the values seen during occasional sphygmomanometric determinations, particularly if an unsettling environment is involved. The detailed differences between occasional determinations and the true average have not been described, however.

Measurements in animals

Arterial pressure is usually measured directly using an indwelling catheter and a pressure transducer. This method will produce values that are accurate at the moment that the pressure is recorded; however, the attendant laboratory procedures may be simultaneously causing pressure to fluctuate away from its long-term or true average.

Anesthesia can make a big difference. Pentobarbital anesthesia in the dog increases pressure. Gilmore (348) reported a mean pressure of 127 mm Hg after one hour of anesthesia and 144 mm Hg after four hours. Many studies using anesthetized dogs have reported comparable pressures as control data. In contrast, pentobarbital anesthesia in the rat maintains (162) or decreases (821) blood pressure, usually the latter.

A casual review by the author of reported values for mean arterial pressure in the conscious dog suggests a range from about 95 mm Hg to 125 mm Hg and sometimes greater, depending on the circumstances. In contrast, Cowley and colleagues (192) monitored arterial pressure continuously in normal dogs and found the mean arterial pressure to be 102 mm Hg.

Pressure has been measured both directly and indirectly in the rat, making this species very popular in blood pressure research. In the late 1930's, sphygmomanometric methods that used the rat's very accessible tail were developed by Byrom and Wilson (132) and Williams, Harrison, and Grollman (988). Only systolic pressure could be measured however. Sobin (886) showed that there was a significant pressure drop along the tail, 4.5 mm Hg per cm of tail under normal conditions, and that an artificially low pressure would be recorded if the tail artery was less than maximally dilated. Rats were heated to produce the requisite vasodilation.

The accuracy of this method, the tail-cuff method, has been examined. Systolic pressures via tail cuff have been compared to pressures recorded from indwelling cannulae and the correlation was found to be very good (754). There also appears to be little difference in normal rats between the tail-cuff systolic pressure and the true mean arterial pressure as determined by indwelling catheter and long-term monitoring (128), (699). But again, the environmental influences in effect when the measurements are made, including restraint and heating, may at times dislodge blood pressure from its usual value. For instance, Bunag (128) found that rats thought to have renal hypertension showed a tail-cuff systolic pressure of 185 mm Hg when restrained and heated, a mean pressure of 171 mm Hg via cannula during the tail-cuff procedure, and a mean pressure of only 115 mm Hg via cannula when monitored over a longer period with minimal restraint. Similarly, Norman and Coleman (699) recently reported that baroreceptor denervated rats showed a tail-cuff systolic pressure of 165 mm Hg when restrained and heated, a mean pressure of 150 mm Hg via cannula when under restraint, and a mean pressure of only 123 mm Hg via cannula when monitored over 24 hours with minimal restraint.

Thus, a fundamental problem keeps reappearing in both the clinic and laboratory: While the individual methods being used may be accurate _per se_, unsuspected or poorly understood environmental and laboratory influences can produce values that are considerably different than the true average arterial pressure.

NORMAL vs. ABNORMAL ARTERIAL PRESSURE LEVELS

The concept of a "normal" pressure remains elusive. Arterial pressure varies from minute to minute as a function of physical and mental activity, as discussed above. Values taken over the longer term are more consistent, however, particularly if short-term variations and measurement artifact have been accounted for. But, we can also expect to find longer-term trends that are linked to age, gender, dietary habits, body weight, and genetic background -- as discussed in the next chapter. In spite of the problems associated with the meaning of "normal," the upper limits of normotension and lower limits of hypertension have been arbitrarily defined to help in categorizing those persons with the highest pressures and, consequently, the greatest chance of developing cardiovascular complications. The World Health Organization (30) defines as normal those pressures which have a systolic component equal to or less than 140 mm Hg _and_ a diastolic component equal to or less than 90 mm Hg. Hypertension includes systolic pressures equal to or greater than 160 mm Hg _or_ diastolic pressures equal to or greater than 95 mm Hg. Cases that fall in between are labelled "borderline" hypertension. No provision has been made for categorizing subnormal pressures.

Curiously, there are no comparable conventions for defining normotension and hypertension in experimental animals, even though many different species are used extensively in blood pressure research. Many experimentally-produced pressure increases are large enough so that there is little controversy over whether or not hypertension has been produced. In other instances, however, induced pressure changes are not very large. Therefore, at the discretion of individual authors, pressure increases from 70 mm Hg to 90 mm Hg in the rabbit and from 120 mm Hg to 170 mm Hg in the rat might both be described as transitions from normotension to hypertension. This ambiguity is probably not very important when studies focus solely on the mechanisms of blood pressure control. But, it is probably very important when the morbidity and mortality of hypertension are being studied in the laboratory.

UNITS OF PRESSURE

Pressure is defined as force per unit area and one would expect that values for arterial pressure would be reported in scientifically correct units. But, that has not been the case to date. The physical units of "mm Hg" and "cm H2O" are length while "atmosphere" is a representation of pressure that is devoid of physical units. The reason for this diversity and lack of rigor is that reporting is often closely wedded to the type of measuring instrument in use - i.e. mm Hg from the mercury manometer. The cost of this convenience is that units such as "mm Hg" and "atmosphere" are awkward at best when used in comprehensive mathematical calculations.

The International System of Units (SI) is metric in nature and defines pressure in terms of the Pascal (abbreviated Pa). The Pascal is named after Blaise Pascal (born 1623 - died 1662) a French mathematician, scientist, and religious activist. Pascal, in addition to making fundamental contributions to mathematics (he was one of the founders of probability theory) and constructing an adding machine (in the 17th century !), first characterized the uniform propagation of pressure through liquid in a closed vessel -- thereby formulating Pascal's law.

The genesis of the physical unit "Pascal" is as follows. The basic unit of mass in the SI system is the kilogram. Force is equal to mass times acceleration and the units of force are therefore kilograms times meters per second squared. This is a Newton. Pressure is equal to force per unit area and the units are Newtons per square meter. This is a Pascal. One mm Hg is equal to 133.3 Pa.

Use of the Pascal produces large numerical values for arterial pressure but this inconvenience has been circumvented by the use of the "kiloPascal" which is abbreviated kPa. One mm Hg ia equal to .133 kPa and this approach to reporting arterial pressure should come into use as fast as the inertia of tradition will allow. In the SI system, the traditionally normal arterial pressure of 120 mm Hg systolic / 80 mm Hg diastolic becomes 16.0 / 10.6 kPa. Similarly, 1 cm H2O is equal to 98.1 Pa or .0981 kPa.

Currently many scientific journals are encouraging the reporting of pressures in kPa, especially if paired with second values in more traditional units. Lippert and Lehmann (593) have recently provided us with a complete description of the International System of Units and the transition that is currently under way in medicine and medical science.

CHAPTER 3

BLOOD PRESSURE IN HUMANS AND EPIDEMIOLOGY

Arterial pressure in humans, reported using systolic and diastolic values, is said to by typically around 120/80 mm Hg. But, specific deviations from the norm have been catalogued, often using studies of large numbers of subjects. Pressure increases steadily with age, except in those societies that have a very low sodium consumption. Reducing the dietary sodium intake in subjects with hypertension will decrease their pressure somewhat. Obesity is associated with increased pressure in children and adults; conversely, weight loss decreases pressure. Children of parents with high blood pressure will tend to have a higher pressure also, and vice versa. This appears to be partly genetic and partly environmental. Curiously, the physiological mechanisms underlying all of these empirical relationships remain unknown.

ARTERIAL PRESSURE vs AGE

A study of 74,000 subjects in the United States by Masters and colleagues (626) provides the following normal values for arterial pressure.

ARTERIAL PRESSURE (mmHg) IN THE UNITED STATES

	Male		Female	
Age	Systolic	Diastolic	Systolic	Diastolic
16	118	73	116	72
18	120	74	116	72
20-24	123	76	116	72
25-29	125	78	117	74
30-34	126	78	120	75
35-39	127	80	124	78
40-44	129	81	127	79
45-49	130	82	131	81
50-54	134	83	137	83
55-59	138	84	138	83
60-64	142	84	144	85

This study and many others, such as (811) and (627), have documented an increasing systolic and diastolic pressure with advancing age. An exception has been found in instances in which sodium intake is very small, as described below.

VARIABILITY

The variability of arterial pressure can be illustrated graphically. If an adequately large number of samples is available, a graph of the frequency of occurance of each pressure (on the ordinate) vs. the pressure itself (on the abscissa) produces a histogram that will usually show that blood pressure is distributed in approximately a normal or Gaussian fashion, being slightly skewed toward the high pressure end. If the distribution is suitably close to normal, it can be accurately described with only two parameters: mean value and standard deviation.

Referring again to the extensive data of Masters etal (626), the variability of systolic and diastolic pressures has been calculated and the data show increasing variability with age. Very roughly, between the ages of 16 and 60, the standard deviations of systolic and diastolic pressure increase from 12 to 22 mm Hg and from 9 to 13 mm Hg respectively. Using the definition of standard deviation, 68% of all subjects can be expected to have pressures inside of these numerical distances from the average normal pressure and 95% of all subjects can be expected to be within twice these limits.

MALES vs FEMALES

The data tabulated above shows that there is little difference in arterial pressure between men and women. Females have slightly lower pressures than males when young. Relatively rapid increases with age abolish these differences and pressures actually appear to be slightly higher in women beyond the age of 60.

ARTERIAL PRESSURE vs SODIUM INTAKE

Two approaches have been used to study the relationship between blood pressure and habitual dietary salt intake. One has been to determine the average pressure and average sodium intake in a population and then to compare these values with comparable data from other populations. The second approach has been to measure individual pressures and intakes within a population to see if a significant pressure - salt intake correlation might emerge. Sodium intake is usually estimated by measuring the amount of sodium excreted in the urine over 24 hours.

Comparisons made between populations

Individuals in industrialized or acculturated societies consume around 200 mmol (mEq) of sodium per day. A variety of studies of populations in isolated and relatively remote areas have provided examples of a much lower sodium intake than this. A low prevalence of hypertension was observed in each instance -- in the Solomon islands (737), Rarotonga and Pukapuka (773), the highlands of New Guinea (871), the Yanomamo Indians at the Brazilian-Venezuelan border (712), and many other comparative locations.

Oliver and colleagues (712) found that the Yanomamo Indians consumed only 1 mmol of sodium per day. Compared to the "normal" values for pressure tabulated above, arterial pressure was low in this society and it remained low throughout life, as summarized in the following table.

ARTERIAL PRESSURE (mmHg) IN THE YANOMAMO INDIANS

	Male		Female	
Age	Systolic	Diastolic	Systolic	Diastolic
0-9	93	59	96	62
10-19	107	67	105	64
20-29	108	69	100	63
30-39	106	69	99	63
40-49	107	67	98	62
50+	100	64	106	64

In contrast, regions with high sodium intake have been shown to have a high prevalence of hypertension. The study of Sasaki (826) in Japanese populations is often used as an example.

There are many features in addition to sodium intake that distinguish these different populations -- including many other aspects of the diet, typical occupations, lifestyle and affluence, physical activity, and so forth. Any or all of these factors could have a strong influence on blood pressure; as of now, they have not yet been systematically verified or ruled out.

Epidemiological studies have shown that a low sodium intake is often accompanied by high potassium intake and the potassium in these instances may be contributing to the prevention of hypertension. Several studies in the 1920's and 30's reported that a large potassium intake would lower blood pressure in hypertensive subjects (3), (639), (772). A similar effect has been seen in experimental animals (51), (207), (641).

Comparisons made within populations

Attempts to show a positive correlation between blood pressure and sodium intake using individual observations within a population have met with limited success at best (838). Joosens and colleagues (490) found a positive salt - pressure correlation in a European study. But many others, such as Miall (646), have not been able to demonstrate a significant correlation.

There are several reasons why this correlation, if it does exist, might be difficult to demonstrate. One is that salt consumption, possibly excessive at the beginning, may decrease because of suppressed sodium appetite as hypertension becomes fully developed. This was suggested by Green and colleagues in 1954 (365) and the more recent data of Berglund etal (70) supports the idea. Adding observations showing high pressure and normal or low salt intake to a potentially significant positive correlation would raise havoc.

Genetic factors could also produce problems. Selective inbreeding has been used to produce strains of rats that either become uniformly hypertensive with increased sodium intake or remain uniformly normotensive with increased intake (203). In a heterogeneous human population, this genetic influence could produce individual observations of high intake and normal pressure or vice versa that would tend to obscure other underlying relationships.

A third problem concerns methodology. Estimates of chronic sodium intake are usually derived from 24-hour urine collections. Daily values, however, are highly variable. Langford and Watson (558) found that short- and long-term urine collections as estimates of sodium intake were not highly correlated. Liu *etal* (595), (596) have recently analyzed this problem and determined that finding a salt intake - blood pressure correlation using single 24-hour samples is not very likely. They concluded that fourteen consecutive day-to-day samples would be more suitable. Cooper *et al* (188) recently followed this strategy and found that blood pressure was proportional to sodium excretion in a group of 74 children when 7 consecutive 24-hour collections were used. No other studies using long-term collections have been reported.

USING SODIUM RESTRICTION TO TREAT HYPERTENSION

The decreased prevalence of hypertension in societies having a low salt intake suggests that sodium restriction might be effective in treating hypertension. This was one of only a few alternatives before the advent of modern antihypertensive therapy, as reviewed by Chapman and Gibbons (144). Kempner (506) showed that a diet consisting of rice, fruit, and virtually no salt was effective in lowering blood pressure in some instances. Many additional studies, such as (116), (238), (250), (683), and (973), confirmed that blood pressure would generally fall when sodium intake was reduced to about 10 mmol per day or less.

A salt-poor diet is not particularly tasty. Pickering (761) comments:

> "Kempner's rice-fruit diet is intolerable to most. But there are a few, who perhaps would have been hermits or martyrs in a previous age, who love the near military discipline and self denial. They are not the kind of patients who like to have me as their doctor."

Less extreme sodium restriction is a more realistic objective but it may also be less effective. Moser (665) has suggested that anything less than severe restriction is not effective. More recent studies have shown small but consistent decreases in pressure with moderate restriction. Parijs and colleagues (742) found that systolic and diastolic pressures fell 8 and 4 mm Hg respectively when sodium intake was halved. Morgen *etal* (662) recently reported somewhat greater decreases over two years with even more moderate restriction.

Zealous dietary restriction is often effective in lowering blood pressure in hypertensives, but it has not been proven to be a practical approach to antihypertensive therapy. Moderate restriction, on the other hand, probably will not produce acceptable pressure reduction in those patients with more severe hypertension. However, moderate sodium restriction in conjunction with pharmacological therapy might prove to be a useful combination.

ARTERIAL PRESSURE vs BODY WEIGHT

The results of a large number of studies over the last six decades have been consistent: on the average, those with the greatest excess of body weight have the highest blood pressure (419), (462), (500), (579). Stated another way, hypertension is more prevalent in the obese than in those with normal or subnormal body weights -- roughly 1 1/2 to twice as prevalent (890). Additional weight gain in adults may be more closely linked to hypertension than obesity that has continued since childhood (869). Weight reduction is often, but not always, associated with a blood pressure decrease (53), (298), (624), (822), (922). Chiang, Perlman and Epstein (149) have provided a comprehensive review of these relationships.

The physiological mechanisms connecting blood pressure control and body weight are not clear. Expanded blood volume and cardiac output have been reported (7). But, conventional procedures for analysis cannot be readily applied to this data. Normal comparisons are often made on a per-unit-weight basis when small differences in weight must be taken into account. In the case of obesity, large variations in body weight and body composition are under consideration and it is difficult at best to assign "normal" and "abnormal" physiological labels to values that themselves are poorly understood functions of body weight and composition.

Whyte (984) has suggested that cardiac output might exceed the dimensional capacity of the aorta in obesity, resulting in an elevated aortic pressure. This is not likely, however, since the aorta can normally accomodate large increases in blood flow at normal or even reduced arterial pressure during peripheral vasodilation. The dimensions of major arteries are probably less important than the resistance to blood flow offered by the arterioles.

Changes in sodium balance may be important in the blood pressure decreases that accompany weight loss. Natriuresis is observed when caloric restriction is initiated (27), (889). Dahl and colleagues (208) argued that the decreased sodium intake that accompanies caloric restriction is a very important component of the hypotensive response. But Reisen etal (790) have recently shown that weight reduction without decreases in dietary sodium intake is also effective in lowering arterial pressure. The matter of calories vs. sodium is not fully resolved; it may be that improved sodium excretion has a stronger influence on blood pressure than the prevailing dietary intake during weight loss.

Young and coworkers may have the explanation. They have recently reported that sympathetic nerve activity is inhibited by fasting (1005), (1006) and this in turn could have a beneficial effect on both vascular tone and sodium balance.

BLOOD PRESSURE AS AN INHERITED TRAIT

Platt observed nearly identical pairs of blood pressures in a small group of hypertensive, identical twins that came to his attention (764). He later postulated:

> "The facts at present known could be explained by the action of a single gene, with incomplete dominance and a frequency of about 0.24, which in the homozygous form gives rise to severe hypertension and in the heterozygous form to moderate elevation of blood pressure."

Pickering (760) rejected this idea and postulated instead that:

> "Arterial pressure is inherited polygenically."

And further, in the etiology of essential hypertension:

> "... inheritance and environment contribute, but environmental factors are more important."

A controversy followed that has not yet been fully resolved. But from the data that is currently available, its not likely that a single gene is responsible for essential hypertension. A better possibility is that the culprit is a few genes in combination with environmental factors.

Many studies have shown that blood pressure aggregates in families. This means that if an individual has a high blood pressure, his or her close relatives (children, parents, siblings) will have a greater than random chance of also having high blood pressure. Similarly, a low pressure will be surrounded by other low pressures. Familial aggregation of blood pressure has raised several important questions that have only been partially answered.

1. What is the quantitative, as opposed to qualitative, contribution of genetic factors?

2. What part of familial aggregation is caused by genetic factors and what part is due to a common environment?

3. What biochemical or physiological mechanisms are involved in implementing genetic influences?

Familial aggregation

Analysis of familial pressure aggregation uses mathematical models of pressure variability. Variability is assumed to be due either to family influences (genetic and shared environment) or to other non-specific influences. This approach has consistently shown strong familial aggregation (55), (92), (414), (432), (482), (647), (764), (1011), (and others). The relationship holds even when young children are studied (55), (56), (91), (432), (442), suggesting genetic rather than environmental influences. But familial aggregation does not directly imply genetic influence; environmental factors could just as well be responsible for some or all of the observed correlation. Therefore, it has not been possible to obtain a quantitative estimate of the genetic influence on blood pressure from these data. Additional methods have been employed to make the distinction.

Genetic vs. environmental influences

It has been very difficult to separate genetic influences from those influences produced by a shared or common environment. Studies to date have utilized spouses, twins, and adopted children.

Spouses share the environmental setting of a family but not the genetic setting and are, therefore, a potentially useful model. Environmental influence would be expressed as a positive blood pressure correlation between husband and wife. Results have been highly variable, showing correlations ranging from none (56), (271), (647) to considerable (424), (941), (992). Therefore, some environmental influence is indicated but other experimental approaches may be more precise.

The origin of pressure differences between monozygotic (identical) twins should be environmental and not genetic; variability between dizygotic (fraternal) twins should be both environmental and genetic. Suitably large groups of twins are not often available for observation, but the results have shown a strong genetic influence on blood pressure (271), (422), (637), (954). Havlik and colleagues (422) studied 7 year-old twins and concluded that about 53% of the variation in distolic pressure and a lesser fraction for systolic pressure is inherited. In studies using 14 year-old twins (637) and adult twins (271) about 60% of the variation in systolic and diastolic pressure appeared to be inherited.

Adopted children share the environment but not the genetic background of the adopting family. Thus, a blood pressure correlation of adopted children with other members of the family can be considered to be due to environmental effects. A long-term study has been taking place in Montreal. Initial results (92), (93) showed no environmental influence on blood pressure. More recent analyses (21), (22) do not agree. About 30% of the variability in pressure has been attributed to genetic factors. However, 11% of the variability in systolic and 20-31% of the variability in diastolic pressure were found in the most recent study to be due to environmental factors. Hence, an environmental component is indicated that is greater than was previously suspected.

The identification of both genetic and environmental influences on blood pressure suggests that genetic factors might predispose an individual to becoming hypertensive; environmental factors such as stress or imprudent sodium intake would then supply the decisive stimuli.

Biochemical and physiological mechanisms

Little is known about the mechanisms participating in the

inherited aspects of blood pressure control. A vast number of traits are under genetic influence, but these traits are not necessarily involved in blood pressure control. Its likely that many spurious connections between genes and pressure will be postulated in the process of making a correct identification.

Several recent studies have shown a genetic influence on autonomic and renal function. The concentrations of two enzymes controlling catecholamine metabolism, catecholomethyltransferase in erythrocytes (35), (36) and monoamine oxidase in platelets (695), (997), have been shown to be under strong genetic control. Julius and Esler (494) summarized the abnormalities seen in patients with borderline hypertension. Arterial pressure, cardiac output, heart rate, and plasma renin activity are all elevated and all can be normalized by autonomic blockade. These young subjects may be part of a peculiar minority, or they may more generally represent an early expression of the genetic factors that encourage the development of essential hypertension. Recently, Falkner and colleagues (267) demonstrated that the response to stress of normotensive children with hypertensive parents was similar to the response of subjects with hypertension, even though the children were not hypertensive at the time of the study. The data suggest that hyperresponsiveness of the autonomic nervous system might be a precursor of the development of hypertension. Grim and colleagues (373), (374) found that close relatives of patients with essential hypertension have higher levels of plasma renin activity and impaired capacity to excrete an infused saline load. Bianchi et al (82) found that the normotensive children of hypertensive parents showed relatively normal renal function except that renal blood flow was elevated. These data suggest that some irregularities in renal performance may precede the development of hypertension.

The way in which the body partitions fluid between the cells and extracellular spaces may also be under genetic control, as recently commented on by Parker (743). Changes in water and electrolyte distribution and vessel wall composition in hypertension are usually thought to be a result of hypertension rather than a cause of it. Postnov et al (768) have observed increased sodium permeability and decreased sodium-potassium ATPase in red cells taken from essential hypertensives. But recently Garay and colleagues (338),(339) have further analyzed sodium and potassium fluxes in erythrocytes.

Sodium-potassium exchange is normal in subjects with secondary hypertension but it is increased in persons with essential hypertension _and_ some of their dependents.

Identification of the biochemical and physiological mechanisms underlying the genetic influences on blood pressure is of great scientific importance, but identification may also be clinically relevant -- those subjects with a particular predisposition to hypertension might benefit from early, moderate changes in diet or lifestyle. Those without such predispositions would not be similarly constrained.

CHAPTER 4

A BRIEF HISTORY OF THE STUDY OF BLOOD PRESSURE CONTROL

Although the seriousness of high blood pressure in humans was appreciated in the 19th centruy, few studies were undertaken to help understand and correct the problem. Then in the 1900's the pace quickened with a rapid succession of advances. First one, then many, reliable experimental models came into general use. The renin-angiotensin system was discovered and characterized in considerable detail. The importance of sodium was investigated using dietary manipulation, epidemiological studies, animal models, and lessons from the management of patients with renal disease who were undergoing chronic hemodialysis. Most recently, the subtleties of neural dysfunction have been studied using sensitive assays for catecholamines.

THE SITUATION BEFORE 1900

Dr. Richard Bright (born 1789 - died 1858) of Guy's Hospital in London characterized a syndrome in 1827 that included albuminuria, atrophied kidneys, hypertrophied heart, vasoconstriction, and apoplexy (stroke). But, there were only minor additional advances in our understanding of hypertension over the next century or so. This was partly due to a lack of suitable experimental models. Wakerlin (967) has provided a concise history.

GOLDBLATT'S TECHNIQUE PRODUCED THE FIRST RELIABLE EXPERIMENTAL MODEL

In 1934, Dr. Harry Goldblatt of Western Reserve University in Cleveland described a hypertension that could be reliably produced in dogs using a clamp placed on the renal artery (353). Initially, in fact, bilateral clamps were used and Goldblatt thought that tightening the clamps produced a renal ischemia that somehow caused elevated arterial pressure.

Previous investigations had evaluated one form of renal

insult or another but with little success. For instance, Lundin and Mark in 1925 (609) showed that reduction of renal mass sometimes led to increased arterial pressure and Dominguez (240) attempted to produce hypertension by injecting uranium. Apfelbach and Jensen (26) injected particles of charcoal into the renal artery. These procedures usually produced severe uremia rather than hypertension.

Goldblatt's procedure produced the first truly reliable experimental model and it has been used most extensively ever since. A connection between the suspected renal ischemia and elevated pressure was provided by the subsequent characterization of the renin-angiotensin system. The following conclusion was a natural one : renal artery constriction leads to increased renin secretion by the kidney and the resultant increase in angiotensin production causes vasoconstriction and hypertension. Subsequent studies have indicated that the complete explanation will not be this simple in the majority of cases.

CHARACTERIZATION OF THE RENIN - ANGIOTENSIN SYSTEM

Although Tigerstedt and Bergman (622), (932) at the turn of the century demonstrated a pressor substance in the kidneys of rabbits, this observation was not utilized further in the years immediately following their report. Then in about 1940 both Page at Indianapolis (733) and Braun-Menendez and colleagues (105) in Argentina independently found a substance of renal origin that by itself was inactive. But, it was either activated by plasma or was involved in a reaction in the plasma that led to the formation of a vasopressor substance.

In the 1950's the vasoactive substance was shown by Skeggs and colleagues in Cleveland (876) and Elliot and Peart in London (256) to be a peptide, angiotensin II, that was formed from another peptide precursor, angiotensin I. The name "angiotensin" was a condensation of "angiotonin" suggested by Page and "hypertensin" suggested by Braun-Menendez (731).

The first chemical determinations of renin and angiotensin were indirect and most difficult. The involvement of the renin-angiotensin system in the genesis of hypertension was supported more by inference than by firm documentation. With accurate determinations of plasma

renin activity now a reality and the development of highly specific blockers to angiotensin converting enzyme and the angiotensin II receptor, it has more recently been demonstrated that the renin-angiotensin system plays less of a role in the genesis of many forms of hypertension than was once suspected. Specifically, high levels of plasma renin and angiotensin seem to be important in some forms of malignant hypertension and in the maintenannce of homeostasis during salt depletion. In most other instances of elevated pressure, plasma levels of renin and angiotensin are close to or even below normal; therefore, a universal (in contrast to specific) role for this humoral system in the genesis of hypertension seems doubtful at the present time. There has been a shift in the emphasis of research to other physiological properties of angiotensin, including the stimulation of thirst, steroidogenesis, and the effects of angiotensin on renal salt and water excretion.

THE BODY'S SALT AND WATER STORES ARE SHOWN TO BE IMPORTANT IN THE GENESIS OF HYPERTENSION

Before the advent of modern antihypertensive therapy, Kemper (506) showed that a drastic reduction in dietary sodium intake would lower blood pressure in hypertensive subjects. Further, a variety of epidemiological studies over the past several decades have shown that populations with a low dietary sodium intake have a low prevalence of hypertension. The advent of chronic hemodialysis for large numbers of patients with end-stage renal disease has presented an opportunity to gain further insight into the role of sodium in the control of blood pressure. Many of these patients show a blood pressure which is sensitive to fluid volume changes. Ultrafiltration during hemodialysis lowers blood pressure; indiscriminate salt and water intake raises blood pressure. These studies point to sodium as an important component in blood pressure control, but they do not indicate what mechanism or mechanisms might be involved.

In 1963 Borst and Borst-de Geus (98) argued that salt and water retention by the kidneys would lead to a tendency for increased cardiac output. But, this tendency would be rebuffed by the capacity of the tissues to maintain normal blood flow. The ultimate result would be elevated pressure and vascular resistance with normal flow. They used these concepts in analyzing the hypertension that occurred in some of their patients who consumed large amounts of licorice; these patients showed overt signs of fluid retention.

Ledingham and Cohen (565) added that if an autoregulatory vascular response was part of the genesis of hypertension, then a transient exchange between blood flow and resistance should be observed. They postulated that flow changes should precede resistance changes and demonstrated this during the pressure decrease that follows unclamping the renal artery in a group of hypertensive animals with renal artery stenosis (564). Since that time the concept has been applied to several other forms of hypertension including salt-loading after subtotal nephrectomy (168).

Actually, two separate concepts are involved in this interpretation of blood pressure control. The first is that arterial pressure will rise to whatever level is necessary to maintain salt and water balance. Either increased salt intake or decreased renal excretory capacity could necessitate a pressure change; it was the latter in Borst's patients. The second concept is that increased vascular resistance, rather than increased blood flow, will supply the needed pressure increase. Vasoconstriction will be generated by a sequence of events that starts with retention of salt and water, is followed by increased cardiac output, and ends with autoregulatory vasoconstriction. This explanation of long-term blood pressure control has been formalized in the past two decades by Guyton and colleagues (391), (393).

RECENT STUDIES IMPLICATE THE CENTRAL NERVOUS SYSTEM

There has been a strong feeling for some time that the nervous system is involved in long-term blood pressure control and that increased autonomic activity might produce chronic hypertension. Smithwick (882) for instance undertook a number of sympathectomies in patients with essential hypertension in an attempt to bring pressure down. We also know that pheochromocytoma is associated with hypertension and increased blood levels of epinephrine and norepinephrine. Surgical removal of the responsible tissue or administration of drugs that interfer with the function of catecholamines will promptly lower blood pressure. But, the role of the autonomic nervous system in other clinical situations and experimental models has remained for the most part speculative over the years.

Several recent developments have rekindled an interest in the connection between the nervous system and blood pressure. Highly sensitive assays for plasma catecholamines are now available (258). These assays have detected small but potentially significant elevations of plasma catecholamine levels in some hypertensive patients and some experimental models. Further, drugs that interfere with central and peripheral autonomic function can often lower blood pressure. It has recently been shown that injection of 6-hydroxydopamine, an agent that destroys sympathetic nerve endings, prevents many forms of experimental hypertension.

> The transition then appears to have been from (1) a search for a renal pressor substance to (2) an interest in dietary sodium and the excretory capability of the kidney to (3) a renewed interest in the nervous control of blood pressure. The current challenge is to reconcile all of the relevant observations, past and present, and to produce an explanation for blood pressure control that is both contemporarily and historically sound.

CHAPTER 5

EXPERIMENTAL HYPERTENSION

While there are many different approaches to the study of the control of arterial pressure, many current research programs are focusing on the homeostatic responses of experimental animals as some intervention is used to induce hypertension. The potential for statistically adequate data groups, valid control data, and reproducibility are attractive scientific features that are sometimes hard to obtain in clinical protocols. Experimental animal models can be roughly grouped according to five types of interventions : the kidney is insulted, sodium balance is upset, normal neural function is interrupted, selective inbreeding raises blood pressure, and humoral vasoconstrictors are infused.

USING EXPERIMENTAL HYPERTENSION TO UNDERSTAND BLOOD PRESSURE CONTROL

The control of arterial pressure is multifaceted. This complexity has encouraged research ranging from studies of the molecular basis of smooth muscle contraction to studies of blood pressure trends in diverse populations. Yet, in trying to analyze the long-term control of arterial pressure, there are only limited opportunities to observe the candidate control processes in action. One approach is to produce hypertension in laboratory animals and then to make detailed observations of the different components of the subsequent response.

ANIMAL STUDIES vs CLINICAL STUDIES

Although human hypertension is a medical problem of major proportions, rigorous investigation in the clinical setting is more often than not a formidable scientific undertaking. Hypertension in humans can sometimes result from known causes such as renal artery stenosis or steroid secreting tumors, but it usually results from no known cause. Therefore, the majority of patients must be classified as having essential hypertension. This hypertension involves a gradual, insidious rise in blood pressure that can span several decades. Clinical observation of such patients usually gives an indication of the current pathophysiological status of the patient but reveals little about the mechanisms that had been involved in the initial pressure increase or the mechanisms that are currently involved in maintaining the elevated pressure. Further, there are often confounding contributions from an unsuitably small number of subjects, diversity of (and incomplete) histories, lack of proper control subjects, uncertainties about reproducibility, and other vagaries.

Animal models of hypertension offer some advantages over clinical investigations. Laboratory protocols can be devised in such a way that the experimental animal is observed before the hypertension producing perturbation, immediately after this perturbation, and in the chronic state of well-established hypertension. Such sequential studies and the invasive procedures that are possible have the potential of revealing mechanisms that are not visible in the clinical studies but that are applicable to the human condition. Further, there is usually little difficulty in evaluating reproducibility, obtaining a statistically significant number of observations and obtaining suitable control data.

TYPES OF EXPERIMENTAL HYPERTENSION

Many different species have been used in laboratory investigations. Rats and dogs have been most extensively employed while rabbits, pigs, sheep, mice and non-human primates have also been used by some investigators. A cursory examination of the literature suggests that an innumerable variety of interventions have been used to produce hypertension in these different species. But upon close inspection, it becomes clear that many experimental models share common features in both the type of perturbation used to produce hypertension and the homeostatic response of the animal. This suggests that there is a natural grouping of experimental models. Five categories are suggested :

1. Models that place the blood supply to the kidney in jeopardy. These models are highlighted by renal artery stenosis but the use of other renal insults is also effective. These models are described in Chapters 6

through 8.

2. Models that involve increased salt intake and/or decreased renal performance. Salt *per se* will produce hypertension but decreased excretory capability of the kidneys facilitates the pressure rise. Decreased capability has been produced by surgically decreasing renal mass but mineralocorticoid excess and other maneuvers are also effective. These models are discussed in Chapters 9 and 10.

3. Models that alter neural function. Incapacitating the baroreceptors and producing lesions within the central nervous system are two of many ways that have been used to disrupt the neural control of arterial pressure. These experiments are discussed in Chapter 11.

4. Models that use infused vasoconstrictors. Angiotensin, norepinephrine and vasopressin have all be chronically administered to produce hypertension. These models are discussed in Chapter 12.

5. Models with a strong genetic component. Selective inbreeding has produced many different strains of animals that become hypertensive with time and in the absence of any superimposed experimental perturbations. These models may or may not share common physiological mechanisms and must, therefore, be considered individually. They are discussed in Chapters 13 through 16.

CHAPTER 6

HYPERTENSION CAUSED BY RENAL ARTERY STENOSIS: GOLDBLATT HYPERTENSION

Renal artery stenosis in conjunction with contralateral nephrectomy rapidly and predictably creates a stable hypertension. The renin-angiotensin system is initially activated but renin levels soon return to normal. In many instances body fluids and cardiac output are initially increased but they also return to normal in time. The eventual hemodynamic picture is one of a persistent hypertension with vasoconstriction and normal blood flow. One explanation is that renal artery stenosis initially impairs renal excretion, but that the situation is redressed by fluid retention, increased flows, autoregulatory vasoconstriction, and reestablishment of normal renal perfusion pressure and excretory capability.

Renal artery stenosis with the contralateral kidney left untouched creates a less predictable and less severe hypertension. Plasma renin levels increase markedly after clamping but they then decrease to levels close to, but significantly above, normal in most cases. There is some evidence for fluid retention and the other indicators that imply autoregulatory vasoconstriction, but the data is much less persuasive than in the model with contralateral nephrectomy. The observation that chronic inhibition of angiotensin II formation lowers blood pressure to normal supports an important causal role for the renin-angiotensin system in this model that may be both pressor and antinatriuretic -- involving particularly the intact contralateral kidney.

ONE-KIDNEY vs TWO-KIDNEY MODELS

Partial obstruction of one renal artery is seen clinically and it is usually accompanied by moderate to severe hypertension. Stenosis can be diagnosed radiographically and by comparing the function of the suspect kidney to the contralateral kidney. Surgical repair lowers blood pressure -- usually to normal. There is a comparable experimental model wherein renal artery constriction is produced by an external clamp in larger animals and an external clip in smaller ones. The blood pressure elevation is proportional to the severity of the constriction (571).

Since Goldblatt's initial demonstration in 1934 of the reliability and utility of this method (353), two major variants have been developed. In one case, one renal artery is constricted and the contralateral kidney is removed. This has been called one-kidney Goldblatt hypertension but a recent recommendation is to call it one-kidney, one clip hypertension (735). In the second model, one renal artery is constricted while the contralateral kidney remains untouched. This is called two-kidney Goldblatt hypertension but two-kidney, one clip hypertension is now the recommended name (735) to distinguish this model from the two-kidney, two clip model that is occasionally used. A more suitable name is Wilson-and-Byrom hypertension, recognizing the originators (989). There are striking differences between the one-kidney and two-kidney models and they will be analyzed individually after some preliminary comparisons are made.

Constriction plus nephrectomy is the more predictable and the more popular of the two preparations. Arterial pressure rises rapidly to a value greater than that seen in the two-kidney model and will remain stable at this level for a long time. Pressure will return to normal in the one-kidney model when the constriction is removed but will remain elevated following nephrectomy (302). The one-kidney Goldblatt model has been produced in a wide range of species including cats, dogs, sheep, rabbits and rats.

Blood pressure elevation in the two-kidney model is less predictable, takes longer to obtain, and is not as great as in the one-kidney model. Plasma renin levels are often raised, although the increase in many instances is relatively small. Although the two-kidney model normally shows moderate pressure elevation, it has a tendency to swing into a malignant, accelerated phase of hypertension with very high blood pressure, salt and water loss, high renin levels and poor prognosis. The two-kidney model has been successfully produced in sheep, rabbits and rats but has been only partly successful in the dog.

The two-kidney model is interesting in that total renal function is divided. One kidney is situated beyond a severe constriction and may be underperfused. In contrast, the untouched kidney is perfused at high pressure and is vulnerable to the damaging influence of this pressure. Humoral and excretory functions are no longer shared equally by the two kidneys. The clamped kidney secretes larger than normal amounts of renin and has decreased total excretion while the untouched kidney appears to secrete no renin at all while excreting the greatest fraction of water and electrolytes leaving the body.

Hypertension in both Goldblatt models is characterized by increased arterial pressure and total vascular resistance with normal cardiac output. A number of explanations for the vasoconstriction have been advanced but none are totally satisfactory. At first it was thought that increased blood levels of renin and angiotensin were enough to cause direct vasoconstriction and pressure elevation. But it now appears that this explanation holds only for the first few hours or days of the pressure increase. More subtle effects of angiotensin have been postulated to revitalize the theory. These will be discussed in more detail later. It has also been postulated that the clamped kidney is not able to excrete normal amounts of salt and water and the resultant fluid retention leads to pressure elevations. Fluid retention is often, but not always, seen in the early stages of hypertension -- particularly in the one-kidney model. Over the longer term, fluid volumes are normal and sometimes they have been observed to be below normal -- particularly in the two-kidney model. Other pressor substances coming from the clamped kidney have been considered, as have the absence of vasodilator substances. Recent experiments have brought the nervous system into the picture, possibly in a causal role but more likely in a permissive role. The data available at this time do not give us a full or simple explanation.

ONE-KIDNEY GOLDBLATT HYPERTENSION

The consequences of renal artery constriction plus contralateral nephrectomy have been most extensively studied in the rat and dog. This maneuver raises the arterial pressure from a mean of around 100 mmHg to a mean of between 140 and 160 mmHg over a week or so following clamping. The exact magnitude and time course of the pressure increase depend upon the severity of clamping and the surgical procedures used. Rats, for instance, are often prepared with a loose-fitting clamp that becomes tighter as the animal grows; blood pressure increases gradually.

The renin-angiotensin system

Renal artery constriction causes a marked decrease in renal perfusion pressure (typically to 50 - 60 mmHg), a decrease in renal blood flow, and dilation of the renal vasculature (418). This is accompanied by marked increases in renin secretion; plasma renin activity rises rapidly (388) and reaches values of four or more times normal in about 1 hour (431).

A three- or four-fold increase in plasma renin activity will produce a direct pressor effect of about 20 to 30 mmHg (136). There is no change in the sensitivity of the peripheral vasculature to angiotensin at this time. Angiotensin infusion at a rate that raises plasma angiotensin II concentration to the level observed after renal artery constriction produces a comparable increase in arterial pressure (136). Furthermore, nephrectomy (759),(803) or infusions of angiotensin analog or converting enzyme inhibitor (169),(652) in this very early stage of hypertension completely normalize blood pressure. It can be concluded then that the increase in plasma renin activity just after renal artery constriction fully accounts for the initial increase in blood pressure.

The elevations in plasma renin activity do not persist however. Levels approach normal within a few days to a week (87),(748). In the chronic situation, subnormal levels of plasma renin concentration and plasma renin activity have occasionally been reported. Renal renin content is normal (650),(786),(937).

There is little evidence that angiotensin is playing an important role during the established phase of hypertension. Removing the renal artery clip rapidly leads to normotension (131) while removal of the sole remaining kidney inactivates the renin-angiotensin system but does not decrease blood pressure (302),(759),(803). Similarly, angiotensin analogs and converting enzyme inhibitor cause small acute decreases in pressure (62),(120),(169),(344),(542) that are not much greater than those seen in normal animals. Long-term inhibition of angiotensin formation lowers blood pressure in this model, but not to normotensive levels (62). Hence, it appears that the renin-angiotensin system plays little role in maintaining high pressure in this type of hypertension but that it does have an important role in elevating pressure at the outset.

Hemodynamics

There is evidence of significant but transient fluid volume expansion at the onset of hypertension. A variety of studies have shown increased blood, plasma, extracellular, and interstitial fluid volumes in the weeks following clamping (183),(275),(551),(552),(903),(934).

Volume expansion is occurring as plasma renin activity is falling and it might be postulated that the volume expansion replaces plasma renin activity as the source of elevated arterial pressure. During this time period pressure distal to the renal artery constriction, i.e. renal perfusion pressure, is returning toward normal (37),(278) as is renal vascular resistance and renal blood flow (278). However, a study by Harris and Ayers (418) has indicated that completely normal values might not develop. Chronically, the kidney appears to have relatively normal function.

The fluid volume expansion could contribute to the maintenance of elevated arterial pressure in several different ways. One would involve increased blood volume and increased venous return leading to an increase in cardiac output. The increased cardiac output would then stimulate autoregulatory vasoconstriction. Another possibility is that increased fluid volume or increased exchangeable sodium has a direct effect on peripheral vascular resistance.

Examination of the venous side of the circulation has revealed decreased venous compliance (863); theoretically, this should enhance the hemodynamic consequences of fluid retention. Mean circulatory filling pressure provides a quantitative estimate of the combined effects of blood volume and vascular compliance changes. Increased values for filling pressure have been observed in one-kidney Goldblatt dogs (795) and rats (998).

Bianchi et al (87) measured a variety of hemodynamic variables in conscious dogs following renal artery constriction and found a transient increase in plasma renin activity with fluid volume expansion. These data are summarized on the next page.

RESPONSE TO RENAL ARTERY CONSTRICTION
AFTER CONTRALATERAL NEPHRECTOMY (87)

	Control	Post-Constriction		
		2 Hours	1 Day	3-4 Days
Arterial Pressure (mmHg)	98	125	123	139
Cardiac Output (l/min)	3.84	4.00	4.21	4.62
Total Peripheral Resistance	2010	2678	2620	2623
Heart Rate (beats/min)	93	97	82	93
Plasma Renin Concentration	8	41	30	35
Plasma Volume (ml/kg)	67	72	77	80
ECFV (ml/kg)	329	-	369	371

Although few longer-term data were collected in this study, the increased cardiac output appeared to be replaced by increased peripheral resistance as both blood flow and fluid volumes moved closer to their initial values. The long-term hemodynamic picture is probably one of elevated arterial pressure and vascular resistance with normal blood flow. Early transients suggest that an initial hyperreninemia is replaced by autoregulatory vasoconstriction as the source of the elevated vascular resistance, but the evidence is only indirect. Hypertension produced solely by humoral vasoconstriction would probably be accompanied by decreased, or at best normal, flows and volumes.

Several other investigators have also observed an increase in cardiac output at the beginning on one-kidney hypertension (275),(566),(938). In the studies of Olmsted and Page (714), cardiac output fell with clamping and was subsequently never above normal. Conway (183) found no change in cardiac output.

Neural factors

Traditionally, the nervous system has been thought to be not involved in one-kidney Goldblatt hypertension. Sympatholytic drugs are not particularly effective in lowering blood pressure. Sympathectomy or renal denervation were shown by Collins (173), Goldblatt *et al* (350) and Freeman and Page (313) to have little effect on the onset of hypertension.

The role of the baroreceptors in this particular model has been extensively studied, beginning in 1940. Goldblatt and colleagues (351) discovered that baroreceptor denervation did not change blood pressure in established hypertension. Kezdi and Wennemark (507) and McCubbin (633) observed that the baroreceptors opposed the early increase in blood pressure but that in several days to a week the neural firing pattern of the baroreceptors reverted back to normal. This suggests that in one-kidney hypertension the early buffering of blood pressure elevation is followed by a complete adaptation of the baroreceptors in the blood vessel wall. Similar adaptive responses have been observed in other types of experimental hypertension (20),(702) with the rat showing particularly rapid adaptation to both increasing and decreasing pressures (539),(820).

It appears that the baroreceptors adapt very early in hypertension and thereby play no significant role over the longer term. This view has been supported by the experiments of Liard *et al* (590) who studied the onset of hypertension in both intact and baroreceptor-denervated one-kidney Goldblatt dogs. Pressure rose gradually after renal artery constriction in the intact dogs. Part of the delay can be attributed to baroreceptor inhibition of renin secretion (18). The denervated dogs showed a rapid rise in pressure during the first day after clamping. Eventually, pressure reached exactly the same levels in the denervated and intact dogs. Comparable results have been obtained by Cowley and Guyton (191) in animals made hypertensive by subtotal nephrectomy and salt-loading. The data in total indicate that the contribution of the baroreceptors is consistent from one animal model to another; they slow the onset of hypertension but do not affect the ultimate level of blood pressure.

Several recent observations have rekindled interest in the role of the nervous system in one-kidney Goldblatt hypertension. Firstly, plasma norepinephrine

(210),(528),(788) and norepinephrine turnover (915) have been found to be increased in the one-kidney model but normal in the two-kidney model. If these levels represent spillover of neurotransmitter, they could be symptomatic of a significant adrenergic vasoconstriction. Further, it has been shown that 6-hydroxydopamine injected into the cerebral ventricles completely prevents the elevation in blood pressure (210),(399). This result contrasts with intravenous administration of 6-hydroxydopamine or anti-nerve growth factor which destroy peripheral sympathetic function but do not prevent the development of hypertension (241),(289) with one exception being noted (38). These data in total suggest that there is a neural component that is essential for the development of hypertension in this preparation. A factor or factors may be coming from the brain that are required for salt and water retention by the kidneys and/or smooth muscle contraction in the peripheral vasculature. It is curious that after 6-hydroxydopamine administration, animals with renal artery constriction apparently maintain salt and water balance even though renal perfusion pressure may be as low as 60 mmHg -- a pressure which is normally associated with only minimal amounts of salt and water excretion. The precise mechanisms involved in the neural influence on pressure changes after renal artery constriction are not known.

The influence of salt intake

A low-sodium diet will generally not prevent the development of hypertension in the one-kidney model (668),(682),(799),(893),(928),(937),(938), although Redleaf and Tobian observed a partial antihypertensive effect (784). After hypertension is fully established in this model, sodium restriction does not appreciably lower blood pressure (784) and instead provokes a renin release that can raise plasma renin activity to very high levels.

A sodium-rich diet increases blood pressure only a little and the increased excretory demands placed on the kidney appear to be met with relative ease (701). This response is little different than that shown by the normal animal subjected to the same perturbations (701).

It has been shown in the one-kidney Goldblatt animal that blocking the renin-angiotensin system during the chronic phase of hypertension causes little acute decrease in pressure (344). Further, sodium restriction causes little decrease in pressure but does cause a compensatory renin release (584). Gavras *et al* (344) have demonstrated that a combination of volume *depletion* and angiotensin blockade causes a precipitous fall in blood pressure. Similar results have been observed in normal animals.

One interpretation is that the mechanisms involved in blood pressure control attempt to maintain renal perfusion pressure at normal levels during renal artery constriction. This is achieved when systemic arterial pressure rises enough to offset the pressure drop across the constriction. The arterial pressure increase may normally be supplied by the mechanisms involved in volume homeostasis. But if adequate volume is not available because of sodium restriction or other interventions, then the renin-angiotensin system will come into play to supply the required pressure. When volumes are not adequate *and* the pressor effects of angiotensin are blocked, then blood pressure falls from the hypertensive levels (584).

Miscellaneous factors

Hypophysectomy lowers blood pressure somewhat in this particular model (736),(835) as it does in normotensive and hypertensive animals in general (104),(708); animals tend to fall into poor health after hypophysectomy and do not appear to be robust enough to raise blood pressure above minimal levels except in response to very forceful stimuli. Adrenalectomy with maintenance steroid or salt therapy does not prevent the onset of hypertension (794),(974).

WILSON-AND-BYROM OR TWO-KIDNEY GOLDBLATT HYPERTENSION

Wilson and Byrom (989) showed in 1939 that renal artery constriction with an intact contralateral kidney will cause hypertension in the rat. The arterial pressure typically increases to between 135 and 150 mmHg, which is a little less than in comparable one-kidney animals. In addition, blood pressure changes are relatively more variable and less predictable in the two-kidney model. The mechanisms involved in pressure elevation in this model seem to be more complex than in the one-kidney model, but the variability just described has surely made some contribution to our lack of understanding.

The two-kidney model has been prepared and studied in many species including rats, rabbits, sheep (95), and dogs (99). In dogs, arterial pressure often shows only mild increases (81),(353) or a marked initial increase followed by a return to normal or slightly elevated levels (353),(976). The pressure response may be related to the methods used in producing the constriction. Fekete (272) used complete renal artery ligation. Bounos and Shumaker (99) and Lupu *et al* (611) used a longitudinal rather than focal constriction and reported excellent results. However, the growth of collateral vessels into the renal capsule in dogs can overcome the effects of clamping, leading to reduced pressure (261). Ligation of collateral vessels will re-elevate blood pressure to hypertensive levels (976),(1012). In contrast to this experience with the dog, Siegal and Levinsky (860) found no evidence of collateral development in the rat after renal artery ligation. Because of the problems surrounding the canine preparation, studies in rats and rabbits have provided most of what we know about the two-kidney model.

The renin-angiotensin system

Leenen and colleagues (572) found that moderate hypertension could develop without increases in plasma renin activity. But others have observed, as in the one-kidney Goldblatt model, early increases in plasma renin activity of three or four times normal following renal artery constriction (81),(136),(630). The initial increases in blood pressure can be attributed solely to hyperreninemia as judged from both blocking studies (169) and the experiments of Caravaggi *et al* (136). As in the one-kidney preparation, angiotensin infusions into normal animals that produced blood levels of angiotensin II comparable to those seen in the two-kidney animal also produced pressure increases that were comparable to those seen in the two-kidney animal. Angiotensin has a direct effect on vascular smooth muscle, but this vasoconstriction may be augmented by an elevation in plasma norepinephrine that appears to be of adrenal origin (345).

Renin secretion is increased at the clamped kidney only (740). Perfusion pressure, renal blood flow (976), and glomerular filtration rate on this side are below normal (220),(610) and the kidney is vasodilated. As arterial pressure increases, renal blood flow and glomerular filtration rate in the clamped kidney return toward normal

(220) but may remain somewhat depressed (843). The kidney atrophies (705). Renin stores within the clamped kidney, as measured by renin granularity, increase in the first week or so after clamping (786) and remain doubled (650),(786),(830),(937). The contralateral kidney is perfused at greater than normal pressure right from the start. The renin content on this side falls to very low levels in about two weeks (650),(786),(830),(937).

Although plasma renin activity decreases with time in this preparation, it does not return to normal or below normal but, on the average, remains elevated. Mean values for groups of animals have been reported to be about 1 1/2 to 2 times normal in benign two-kidney hypertension with a range of normal to three times normal being typical (430),(830),(976). These levels of plasma renin activity have only a moderate pressor effect as seen from the acute pressure decrease produced by angiotensin analog or converting enzyme inhibitor. Pressure decreases from 0 mmHg to about half way back to normotension have been reported (120),(138),(169),(342),(542),(612),(976). In some instances the animals under study have been conscious and the buffering effect of the baroreceptors may have prevented larger changes from occurring.

The importance of small increases in plasma renin activity remains controversial. Much larger increases are seen during salt depletion with little change in pressure and little vasoconstriction. On the other hand, chronic blockade of angiotensin formation completely normalizes blood pressure in the two-kidney model (62). Because the immediate pressure decrease with blockade is less than the eventual pressure decrease, some action or actions of angiotensin in addition to direct vasoconstriction are implied.

Non-vasoconstrictor actions of angiotensin have been identified and some time may be required for the full effects of these actions to develop. Angiotensin has been shown to stimulate thirst (297), to have a direct antinatriuretic effect on the kidneys, and to stimulate aldosterone secretion. Singer *et al* (870) and others (233) have observed increased plasma aldosterone concentrations in the two-kidney model. Hence, small increases in plasma renin activity may have important consequences beyond direct vasoconstrictor effects.

Hemodynamics

Evidence that fluid retention has an important role in this preparation is less convincing than in the one-kidney model. Bianchi et al (81) found sequential increases in plasma and extracellular fluid volume in conjunction with increased cardiac output that were reminiscent of their observations in the one-kidney model. However, the pressure increases in the two-kidney dogs were unimpressive. This data is summarized below.

RESPONSE TO RENAL ARTERY CONSTRICTION
WITH THE CONTRALATERAL KIDNEY INTACT (81)

		Post-Constriction	
	Control	1 Day	1 Week
Arterial Pressure (mmHg)	99	112	109
Cardiac Output (l/min)	3.95	4.62	3.65
Total Peripheral Resistance	2076	2136	2518
Heart Rate (beats/min)	96	97	101
Plasma Renin Concentration	8	21	10
Plasma Volume (ml/kg)	70	77	74
ECFV (ml/kg)	353	390	361

Maxwell et al (630) observed increased cardiac output and sodium retention after clamping. Other reports are divided between some fluid retention (551),(572),(630),(656) and no fluid retention (552),(903),(934) in the early phases of two-kidney Goldblatt hypertension. Hence, one is left with the impression that some fluid retention does occur, that it is not a very large amount, and that both the magnitude and the duration of fluid retention are not crisply defined. The relatively gradual increase in pressure that occurs in this preparation may contribute to the lack of certainty.

Simon (863) has observed decreased venous compliance in two-kidney Goldblatt rats. This makes interpretation of volume changes more complicated, while maintaining the possibility that a relative overhydration might develop in the absence of gross fluid retention.

It would be convenient to think that fluid retention increased cardiac output and triggered an autoregulatory response in two-kidney Goldblatt hypertension, but the data now at hand does not justify such a general conclusion. Important trends may be obscurred by the fact that these animals have a tendency to drift into malignant hypertension -- a syndrome characterized by rapidly rising blood pressure, intermittent natriuresis and diuresis, and negative sodium balance.

Neural factors

Studies of the sympathetic nervous system in two-kidney Goldblatt hypertension have produced variable results but, in general, the sympathetics do not appear to have a very important role. Plasma norepinephrine (209),(528),(788) and norepinephrine turnover (915) have been found to be normal. In established hypertension, peripheral sympathectomy will lower blood pressure only temporarily (547),(774). With early peripheral sympathectomy, there is some increase in pressure but hypertension does not develop fully (155). The data is not consistent for central sympathectomy. Injections of 6-hydroxydopamine into the cerebral ventricles does not lower pressure in established hypertension (547), but this procedure has been reported to both prevent (547) and not prevent (209) the development of hypertension.

The importance of the contralateral kidney

Changes in the performance of the contralateral kidney in the early stages of hypertension can probably be considered to be functional changes. In the later stages of chronic hypertension, functional and pathological changes are combined with a high probability that pathology will dominate the overall performance.

The excretion of salt and water by the kidney is highly sensitive to, among other things, changes in perfusing pressure. Studies in isolated, perfused kidneys some two decades ago by Thurau and Deetjen (925), Selkurt (851) and others (499),(635),(859) showed that excretion falls to negligible levels at a perfusing pressure of around 60 mmHg and rises rapidly as perfusing pressure is increased. A more dramatic, but also more difficult to interpret, phenomenon has been observed in the intact animal. When sodium intake is chronically raised or lowered and sufficient time is allowed to permit salt and water balance to be established, large increases in salt and water excretion occur in conjuction with very small increases in arterial pressure (219),(513),(701). In these intact preparations, we can postulate that inhibition of autonomic nervous activity, inhibition of angiotensin formation (219),(513), suppression of aldosterone secretion, and other factors all promote salt and water excretion in excess of those values shown in the isolated, perfused preparation.

These observations indicate that the contralateral kidney has the capability of excreting very large quantities of salt and water when perfused at the levels of pressure that occur in two-kidney Goldblatt hypertension. Excretion should theoretically be great enough to salt and water deplete the animal and to prevent the hypertension from developing. Or, at least this hypertension should evolve in a high-renin, volume-contracted form. But this does not happen: Renin levels are modestly elevated, volume is normal or possibly a little expanded, and total salt-and-water excretion is normal. Split function studies have shown that the contralateral kidney excretes about two-thirds of the total salt and water in the two-kidney preparation (220),(537),(1013). The implication is that there are extrinsic influences operating on the contralateral kidney to suppress its full potential for salt and water excretion.

Angiotensin is antinatriuretic. Infusion of physiological amounts has been shown to decrease salt and water excretion (311),(748),(978). Further, DeClue *et al* (219) countered angiotensin suppression during salt loading by continuous infusion of this peptide. Much higher arterial pressures, and therefore renal perfusion pressures, were needed to achieve a given level of sodium excretion when the suppression of angiotensin formation was overridden.

In 1969, Guyton and Coleman (392) suggested that angiotensin might be responsible for the decreased excretory function in the contralateral kidney. The kidney is renin depleted (650),(786),(830),(937) but it could be under the influence of arterial angiotensin concentrations arising from the renin secretion of the clamped ipsilateral kidney. Micropuncture studies have shown that afferent resistance is increased in the contralateral kidney (843). Zimmerman *et al* (827),(1010) and recently others (461),(625) have shown that acute inhibition of angiotensin formation or angiotensin receptor blockade increases renal blood flow, glomerular filtration, and salt and water excretion in the contralateral kidney, indicating that angiotensin is having some effect on this side. Thompson and Dickinson (924) studied isolated perfused contralateral kidneys from

hypertensive rabbits and found decreased excretion at all perfusion pressures, although it is not clear in this preparation if the depression is functional as described above or due to accumulated vascular damage as described below. In total, it would appear that hypertension is initially maintained in the two-kidney Goldblatt model because the excretory capability of the ipsilateral, clamped kidney is severly depressed by the presence of the clamp and the excretory capability of the untouched contralateral kidney is depressed by angiotensin.

We can use this conclusion to interpret unclamping and nephrectomy studies. Liard found that removing the ipsilateral kidney in the early stages of hypertension results in a fast return to normotension (583). Removing the contralateral kidney results in a further rise in arterial pressure (583),(803). This data is summarized below.

PLETHYSMOGRAPHIC ARTERIAL PRESSURE (mmHg) IN TWO-KIDNEY GOLDBLATT HYPERTENSION FOLLOWING NEPHRECTOMY (583)

		Post-Nephrectomy	
	Control	24 Hrs	5 Days
Clamped Kidney Removed	159	112	
Contralateral Kidney Removed	163	167	173

The blood pressure in the two-kidney model appears to be at the level needed to achieve sodium balance; the requisite pressure is considerably above that required by an animal with a single normal kidney and it is below that required by an animal with a single kidney plus renal artery constriction.

The ipsilateral kidney is protected in a sense because of the pressure drop that occurs across the stenosis. The contralateral kidney on the other hand is left fully unprotected and it is vulnerable to the damages induced by increased arterial pressure, as are the cerebral, coronary, and other regional vascular beds. Vascular damage, falling under the general heading of nephrosclerosis, develops and this damage in turn depresses excretory function in a previously normal kidney. It has been reported that in time this kidney is capable of sustaining hypertension alone and that it recovers its capacity to secrete renin. Wilson and Byrom (990), Floyer (301), and later Thurston <u>et al</u> (926) showed that in the later stages of hypertension removing the clamped kidney leads to only partial restoration of normal blood pressure in most instances. Unclipping sometimes normalizes blood pressure (138),(926) but Floyer (301) found examples in which unclipping did not restore blood pressure to normal levels. If the previously clipped kidney was fully protected from the development of nephrosclerosis, we would expect it to be capable of normalizing blood pressure just as it does when unclipped in the early stages of hypertension. But if the contralateral kidney is damaged, there may be a reversal of roles for the two kidneys from their initial situation; the contralateral kidney in these instances might be capable of producing some elevation in pressure even in the presence of a rejuvenated, unclipped, and presumably fully functional ipsilateral kidney. Unclipping plus contralateral nephrectomy completely normalizes blood pressure (301).

There is some relevant clinical data. Several isolated reports have indicated that in unilateral renal artery stenosis in human beings, surgical repair of the stenosis would not normalize pressure. It appeared that the contralateral kidney was then the culprit and ipsilateral surgical repair was combined with contralateral nephrectomy (!) to produce normotension (654),(631),(923).

The influence of salt intake

Several different inquiries into the sensitivity of the two-kidney Goldblatt preparation to changes in sodium intake have shown that increased intake raises blood pressure while decreased intake has little effect on pressure. In one instance, Miksche and colleagues (650) reported that severe sodium restriction prevented hypertension in the two-kidney model but not in the one-kidney model, although this demonstration of the potency of sodium restriction in the two-kidney model has not been repeated (295),(682),(784),(928),(937).

Swales *et al* (904) have characterized the two-kidney model as renin-dependent and the one-kidney model as sodium dependent. Volume was altered by peritoneal dialysis and saline infusion; the two-kidney hypertensive rat did not show pressure changes while the one-kidney rat did (902). Although acute changes in volume status in anesthetized animals are not strictly comparable to longer-term dietary considerations, these results indicate that there may be some sodium-related differences between the one- and two-kidney models.

In total, both one- and two-kidney Goldblatt animals seem to be able to maintain sodium homeostasis during large increases and decreases in dietary sodium intake with little change in arterial pressure.

Malignant hypertension

Mohring and others have described malignant hypertension in the two-kidney Goldblatt rat in detail. Malignancy is seen most often when a tighter than normal clip is placed on the renal artery (572). Pressure gradually creeps upward until a critical value of 170 or 180 mmHg mean pressure is reached (656). At this point, the contralateral kidney becomes a salt-losing kidney, large amounts of salt and water are lost into the urine (659), fluid volumes become contracted, plasma renin activity rises to a very high level (659), weight loss is observed, vasopressin (658) and aldosterone (572) are increased, and a poor prognosis develops (659). In a recent study, Schomig *et al* (841) reexamined the problem and concluded that pressure-induced volume contraction can occur over a wide range of pressures rather than at a particular critical pressure.

Sheep have also shown excessive sodium loss with very high renin levels during severe hypertension (95).

In malignancy, the clamped kidney may be evolving into more of an endocrine organ than an excretory organ. The secretion of large amounts of renin, with resultant plasma angiotensin increases, might produce a greater vasoconstrictor effect in the systemic circulation than antinatriuretic effect on the contralateral kidney. Pressure-induced natriuresis by the contralateral kidney would follow; contracted fluid volumes would provoke even greater renin release and a vicious cycle would result.

Mohring and colleagues (659) found that administration of saline will break up the vicious cycle, presumably by volume expansion and inhibition of renin release. Added salt is often a hypertensive agent but in this topsy-turvy preparation it has temporarily become a hypotensive agent. Arterial pressure falls. This response will probably not continue in perpetuity but benefits over a week or two have been reported. Chronic feeding of a salt-rich diet or saline has been shown to increase mortality and accelerate vascular damage (244).

These observations are consistent with the idea that the clamped kidney has the bulk of secretory function in the malignant two-kidney model while the unclamped kidney has the bulk of the excretory function. These two functions may be connected by renin of ipsilateral origin producing angiotensin that eventually has a contralateral effect. Further, there may be a fine balance between the antinatriuretic hormonal influences and natriuretic pressure influences; these two in opposition place the contralateral kidney in a crucial position in this model.

Hyperreninemia and volume contraction seem to be more detrimental in malignant hypertension than the pressure increase _per se_. Excision of the _contralateral_ kidney has been shown by Dietz _et al_ (231) to interrupt the vicious cycle of malignant hypertension. Stable hypertension and decreased mortality result, even though the mean arterial pressure is _greater_ after nephrectomy than it was in the previously malignant animal.

REVERSAL OF GOLDBLATT HYPERTENSION

Data collected during the reversal of hypertension might be used to understand its genesis. Blood pressure may be partly or completely normalized by removal of the clip in the one-kidney model and removal of the clip or ipsilateral kidney in the two-kidney model. If renin levels are high, they will fall. Natriuresis may occur.

Liard (584),(591) and others (804) have followed sodium excretion with unclipping in the one-kidney model. Unclipping led to natriuresis and a blood pressure decrease. Unclipping plus ureteral ligation prevented the natriuresis and pressure decrease. Giving a diuretic to the clipped animal did not decrease pressure but it did stimulate renin secretion; pressure decreased with subsequent nephrectomy in proportion to the previous sodium loss. These observations suggest that pressure is normalized after unclipping by a combination of an increase in sodium excretion and decrease in plasma renin activity -- if renin is elevated. Conflicting evidence comes from Funder _et al_ (333) who unclipped one-kidney Goldblatt sheep. Arterial pressure returned to normal after one day or so but no changes were seen in either plasma renin activity or sodium excretion.

The two-kidney model might also be expected to show a brisk natriuresis with unclipping, but most reports claim little or no natriuresis (920). Thurston et al (927) have seen a positive, rather than negative, sodium balance in the week after unclipping.

Ledingham and Cohen (564) observed that cardiac output and arterial pressure decreased after unclipping before peripheral resistance fell, but Hallback-Norlander and colleagues (411) observed pressure and resistance decreases with an increase in cardiac output. Krieger and colleagues (540) found a decrease in cardiac output with both unclipping and sham unclipping.

Lucas and Floyer (604) found that blood pressure fell rapidly with unclipping before a natriuresis had begun. They thought that a shift of plasma to the interstitium had occurred; this would in effect shrink vascular volume without any change in external balance. The underlying idea is that a substance with hypotensive action and of renal origin is released when the renal artery is unclipped.

Others have sought evidence for a renal hormone with vasodepressor action. Floyer (302) and later Muirhead and Brooks (671) found that blood pressure decreased rapidly with unclipping even though the ureter had been sutured into the vena cava. No urine was lost from the body and humoral factors were suggested. But Muirhead and Brooks (671) also found that arterial pressure did not decrease after unclipping if the ureter was simply ligated instead of being placed in the vena cava. It was therefore hypothesized that ureteral ligation increases pressure in the renal medulla and prevents normal release of a hypotensive substance of medullary origin. The hypotensive function of the renal medulla (670) is reviewed more fully in a following chapter. Blood pressure changes in protocols that reroute urine into the vena cava should be interpreted with caution. Vasoactive substances that are normally found only in excreted urine are placed instead in the circulation.

Urine reinfusion or replacement of lost urine with physiological solutions are two techniques that have also been used to prevent negative sodium balance after unclamping. Larger and larger rates of urine flow are observed in these protocols and infusion rates must be increased accordingly. But, arterial pressure decreases (671),(723) even though it seems certain that the body's sodium stores had not been diminished.

The most provocative data comes from acute protocols; but, the normalization of arterial pressure after unclipping is in reality another facet of the long-term process that increased pressure in the first place. A note of caution can be found in the data of Dietz _et al_ (232). They began with hypertensive animals having two kidneys and two renal artery clamps. One clamp was then removed. Natriuresis and normotension followed. But, removal of the clamp had in effect transformed the animal into a standard two-kidney Goldblatt preparation. Arterial pressure would be expected to increase back to hypertensive levels in an experiment of longer duration. Similarly, in hypertensive animals with ureters implanted into the vena cava, arterial pressure decreases rapidly after unclipping but then pressure tends to creep back toward hypertensive levels over the next few days (302). With the data currently available, it is difficult at best to separate acute from chronic mechanisms and to separate the essential aspects from the incidental.

This is a tentative summary of the events that follow renal artery unclamping: Arterial pressure falls more rapidly than it increased. If abnormal, plasma renin activity returns to normal. Sodium excretion increases although this is not absolutely necessary. The kidney appears to release a substance that is active in redistributing body fluids and decreasing cardiac output; it may also have a direct effect on vascular resistance. Therefore, the events that occur during the reversal of Goldblatt hypertension are at least as complex as those that occur at the onset.

CHAPTER 7

HYPERTENSION CAUSED BY OTHER RENAL INSULTS

Various renal injuries have been screened to see if hypertension would result. Two of the most successful: The Page procedure in which the renal capsule is surrounded with an irritating material such as cellophane, and the Grollman procedure in which the renal capsule is compressed by a figure-of-eight ligature. The cause of hypertension and vasoconstriction in these two models remains unclear. Plasma renin activity is not elevated. There is little evidence supporting autoregulatory vasoconstriction. One peculiarity is that unilateral insult must almost always be combined with contralateral nephrectomy before blood pressure will increase. By analogy, the mechanisms involved in the pressure increase may be similar to those that are active in one-kidney Goldblatt hypertension.

PAGE OR PERINEPHRITIC HYPERTENSION

Page in 1939 (729) showed that external compression of the kidney leads to hypertension. This model has been variously called Page hypertension, wrapping hypertension, perinephritic hypertension, or cellophane-wrapping hypertension. In all cases, material is placed around the kidney to prevent further enlargement of the kidney and to irritate and thicken the capsule. This model has been developed in dogs, rabbits and rats using such materials as collodion (a predecessor to modern plastics), cellophane, and gauze soaked in turpentine. Usually, bilateral wrapping or wrapping plus nephrectomy are employed and this suggests that the Page model may resemble the one-kidney Goldblatt model more than the two-kidney Golblatt model.

Lewis and Lee (582) observed increased plasma renin activity in Page hypertension in rabbits, particularly in the first week after wrapping. Other studies have reported normal (135),(484) or low (469) plasma renin activity. The blood pressure decrease with administration of angiotensin analog is unexceptional (299),(469), (484).

The hemodynamics of this preparation have been studied by Ferrario et al (280) in dogs. They found that ipsilateral wrapping with the contralateral kidney left untouched did not elevate blood pressure but produced an increase in cardiac output. Subsequent contralateral nephrectomy produced hypertension and a further increase in cardiac output. Plasma volume neither increased nor decreased. Measurements of mean circulatory filling pressure, an estimate of the effectiveness of blood volume relative to the compliance of the circulation, showed elevated levels. Therefore, relative but not absolute volume expansion had occured in these experiments. These conclusions are in accord with reports of decreased regional venous compliance in Page hypertension (724),(865).

Fletcher et al (300) have studied bilateral wrapping in the rabbit and found, on the contrary, that pressure and resistance increase in parallel while cardiac output decreases over the first few weeks of hypertension. Elevated plasma renin activity might be the cause of the observed vasoconstriction, but this idea is not supported by the observation that infusion of a potent angiotensin antagonist produces little decrease in arterial pressure (299).

Page and Lewis (734) showed that wrapping the kidney with cellophane will produce hypertension in animals on either salt-rich or salt-poor diets. This has been confirmed by Freeman and colleagues (316).

Injection of 6-hydroxydopamine into the cerebral ventricles interrupts central sympathetic function and prevents the development of hypertension in this model (358).

GROLLMAN OR FIGURE-OF-EIGHT LIGATURE HYPERTENSION

Another external renal insult was invented in 1944 by Grollman (378). He tightened a ligature around the capsule of the kidney in a figure-of-eight fashion. The most common approach is to combine a Grollman ligature with contralateral nephrectomy in rats. As in Page hypertension, external compression produces a slowly developing hypertension. Grollman thought that the gradual increase in pressure mimicked the usual clinical course of hypertension and considered this a virtue of his preparation. However, insidious increases of pressure frequently prevent a clear-cut description of the events that are involved in the onset of hypertension.

Exchangeable (381) and total body (367) sodium are increased. Plasma renin activity is probably normal (379). Little additional data is available to help identify the mechanisms involved in the pressure increase.

MISCELLANEOUS INSULTS

In a very early undertaking, Pedersen (749) produced hypertension in rabbits by ligating the renal vein.

Hypertension accompanying pyelonephritis is a clinical entity and an experimental model would be most welcome. Shapiro *et al* (856) repeatedly punctured the kidney with pins to produce inflammation and infection in rats. A mild hypertension resulted though it seems that the model has not proven to be a very useful one.

Many other insults have been tried -- with variable success. Renal anoxia will later produce hypertension (632). Renal irradiation with uranium wasn't successful (240). Microembolization has been produced by charcoal (26), microspheres (296),(525), platelet aggregates (661) and miscellaneous other small particles (9),(661). Glomerular nephritis has been induced using glomerular basement membrane antiserum (332),(852),(887).

Hypertension frequently accompanies renal disease and many animal models have primarily been used to study renal pathology rather than hypertension. Consequently, the available data is more generally relevant to renal disease than to blood pressure regulation. Firm conclusions about specific defects in blood pressure control in these various models are not possible. Unusual models do illustrate, however, that there is a conspicuous renal involvement in most forms of experimental hypertension.

CHAPTER 8

COARCTATION OF THE AORTA

Coarctation of the aorta is a serious, although rather rare, clinical occurance that is ammenable to surgical repair. Experimentally produced coarctation is most useful in that both hypertensive and normotensive tissues are available for study.

As expected, the immediate hemodynamic response to aortic stenosis is a pressure increase above the lesion and a pressure decrease below it. This is followed by a peculiar transition to the chronic state that depends on whether the coarctation is located above or below the origin of the renal arteries. If above, proximal hypertension and distal normotension develop. If below, proximal normotension and distal hypotension are observed. In both cases, renal perfusion pressure returns to about normal and this suggests that some aspect of renal function determines the final outcome.

Almost all clinical and experimental studies have involved lesions above the kidneys, with proximal hypertension and distal normotension. Normal blood flow with vasoconstriction in the upper torso and normal flow with normal resistance in the lower torso have been reported; an autoregulatory response would explain these findings. But, reports of distal vasoconstriction at normal perfusion pressure suggest that a more complex explanation is necessary. Plasma renin activity is usually normal and body fluids, if changed at all, are slightly expanded. In most respects coarctation of the aorta resembles one-kidney Goldblatt hypertension, and the same physiological processes may be involved in both cases.

ACUTE COARCTATION

There are several reasons why coarctation of the aorta cannot be analyzed solely in the simple terms of an increased resistance to blood flow occuring in the aorta. Firstly, coarctation usually occurs at a singular point that impedes blood flow but does not resemble the diffuse arteriolar resistance that occurs elsewhere in the body. Blood flow through an arteriole is believed to be proportional to arterial pressure and the pressure-flow ratio is defined as resistance; the determinants of resistance are incorporated into Poiseuille's law. A discrete constriction shows a different hemodynamic response. Flow through the coarctation is thought to be proportional to the square root of the pressure gradient and the classical concept of resistance to blood flow does not apply. The hemodynamics are described by the orifice equation and the exact relationship between the pressure gradient and flow is a function of the detailed anatomy proximal, within, and distal to the constriction (1002),(1003),(1004). Most notably, the pressure gradient across the constriction increases in proportion to the blood flow through the constriction raised to the second power. Another consideration in coarctation of the aorta is that the eventual hemodynamic picture is not necessarily the same as the initial, acute situation as will be discussed in the next section.

The acute response to small reductions in aortic cross-sectional area is unexceptional. Gupta and Wiggers (387) showed that the cross-sectional area must be reduced down to twenty per cent of the normal area or less before an appreciable pressure gradient (50 mmHg or greater) is created. With a constriction of this severity, mean pressure proximal to the constriction increases as does pulse pressure. The mean and pulse pressure distal to the constriction decrease. Very roughly, the distal pressure decrease is a little larger than the proximal pressure increase (387).

CHRONIC COARCTATION OF THE AORTA

The chronic hemodynamic picture depends on the acute response plus the specific location of the coarctation. Rytand (812), (813) first showed that if the coarctation was above the origin of the renal arteries, proximal hypertension and distal normotension would develop. Conversely, if the coarctation was situated below the origin of the renal arteries, proximal normotension and distal hypotension would develop. Rytand did not measure blood pressure but instead used cardiac hypertrophy as evidence for the presence of hypertension. Goldblatt etal (352) subsequently obtained the pressures that confirmed Rytand's observations. Scott and colleagues (847), (848) followed the time course of the acute to chronic transition in dogs and found that several weeks elapsed before the eventual hemodynamic pattern became fully developed. These data indicate that the kidneys have a very powerful long-term influence in coarctation of the aorta. Renal perfusion pressure is chronically maintained at about normal levels when the coarctation is proximal to or distal to the origin of the renal arteries.

The most common experimental model is one in which the coarctation is located just above the origin of the renal arteries. Severe hypertension develops proximal to the coarctation in the upper half of the body. Increases in plasma renin activity might be suspected to be playing a role, but several different studies have shown that plasma renin activity is within normal limits (42),(44),(955). Futher, chronic inhibition of the renin-angiotensin system in experimental coarctation has been shown to lower blood pressure only slightly (684). Body fluids have been observed to be slightly expanded (42). As emphasized by Alpert <u>etal</u> (13), coarctation resembles one-kidney Goldblatt hypertension in these respects and because all renal tissue is distal to an arterial stenosis. Therefore, the detailed considerations of blood pressure control following renal artery stenosis plus contralateral nephrectomy can probably be applied also to coarctation of the aorta without substantial error.

There are at least two sites of vasoconstriction in coarctation: One is at the primary site in the aorta and the other is in the arterioles within the vascular beds of the upper torso. Freis (318) reviewed the matter in 1960 and cited blood flow studies in the arms of patients with coarctation that showed normal values for blood flow. With normal flow at an elevated perfusing pressure, the calculated vascular resistance in the arms is increased. Freis attributes this to an autoregulatory response but, although this seems to be a reasonable assumption, it has not yet been proven. Blood flow data comes from a rather small number of clinical observations (746),(968) which leaves some room for doubt. But if the data are accurate, coarctation of the aorta proximal to the origin of the renal arteries produces a hemodynamic picture of: Increased arterial pressure proximal to the coarctation, approximately normal values for plasma renin activity and body fluids, and vasoconstriction in the proximal vascular beds.

Nolla-Panades (696) and Bell and Overbeck (60) have reported hemodynamic abnormalities in the lower torso in

rats with coarctation. Hindlimb perfusion studies have demonstrated increased vascular resistance in these beds and increased resistance at maximum vasodilation. It is not known if this abnormality is also present in the intact animal; normal leg blood flow has been reported in several clinical studies (413), (746),(968).

Some other peculiarities have been seen in the lower torso. Hollander etal (444) and Villamil and Matloff (963) originally reported increased sodium and water content in the aorta above the site of coarctation with normal values below the coarctation. These observations suggest that a pressure-induced and secondary change in vessel wall composition occurs in the proximal region. But recently, Pamnani and Overbeck (725), (739) have observed unusual vessel wall composition in the distal and normotensive region. Bevan and colleagues (74),(76) have observed early increases in vessel wall mass and catecholamine content in tissues located proximal to the coarctation. Vascular responsiveness to norepinephrine or sympathetic stimulation was also increased. In long-standing coarctation, the only remaining abnormality was increased wall mass (75). Curiously, early in coarctation the responsiveness to norepinephrine is also increased in veins located below the coarctation. These observations remain unexplained; but, the observed changes have not been particularly large and it may be that a neural or circulating humoral factor is having a mild general vascular effect.

COARCTATION OF THE AORTA IN HUMANS

Coarctation in humans is usually congenital. It occurs with a great variety of manifestations and is often accompanied by defects in the heart and other great vessels (141), as reviewed by Cheitlin (147). Diversity has hindered systematic scientific study of the clinical situation.

Endocrine and hemodynamic factors are similar to those reported for experimental coarctation. Plasma renin activity is usually close to normal (13),(620) although increased renin levels have also been reported (268). Plasma and extracellular fluid volume may be expanded (13),(664). Renal blood flow and glomerular filtration rate may be normal or low, as discussed by Van Way and colleagues (955). Coarctation and the associated proximal hypertension can cause significant increases in the demands placed on the heart and heart failure can develop.

In 1945 Crafoord and Nylin (196) and Gross (385) showed that coarctation could be surgically corrected and, subsequently, children are routinely operated on at a young age with favorable results. Immediately after resection, arterial pressure often rises to dangerously high levels and acute antihypertensive therapy is required. But the hypertension is temporary and normotension is subsequently seen in both the upper and lower torso. Increased plasma catecholamines (61), (800) and increased plasma renin activity (800) have been implicated in this "paradoxical" hypertension.

Surgical correction decreases long-term mortality but not all of the way to normal (896). There is still a significant incidence of cardiovascular disease that might be related to concomitant cardiovascular problems as well as lingering effects of the coarctation *per se*. Frequently a small residual pressure gradient across the coarctation is observed that can become very much larger during exercise (312). Samanek and colleagues (823) and Sivertsson *etal* (872) have reported a continuing vasoconstriction in the upper extremity of subjects many years after successful surgical corrections. This leaves open for debate the question of whether or not the early influences of coarctation on the microvasculature are subsequently reversible.

Animal studies indicate that coarctation is particularly resistant to long-term antihypertensive therapy (684).

CHAPTER 9

HYPERTENSION DUE TO EXCESSIVE DIETARY SODIUM AND/OR ADRENAL STEROIDS

When a large amount of salt is given acutely, it is rapidly excreted by the kidneys. When the same amount is administered chronically, it usually produces a gradual but steady increase in arterial pressure which might be due to declining kidney function. The hypertensive process can be quickened and exacerbated by combining a high sodium intake with partial nephrectomy or added mineralocorticoids.

A partial nephrectomy that decreases renal mass to one-half or one-third of normal has little effect on pressure. But hypertension is rapidly produced when partial nephrectomy and salt loading are combined. Similarly, mineralocorticoids alone cause pressure increases in some but not all instances. The combination of mineralocorticoids plus salt excess is a much more reliable way to produce hypertension.

These models share some common features. Sodium is retained. The renin-angiotensin system is suppressed. In addition to exchangeable sodium, blood volume and cardiac output are sometimes increased -- particularly during early transients. Total peripheral resistance is elevated in the established phase of hypertension. The cause of the vasoconstriction is not settled, but candidate mechanisms include autoregulatory vasoconstriction, increased activity of the sympathetic nervous system and a direct effect of sodium on vascular smooth muscle.

SODIUM, RENAL FUNCTION AND STEROIDS

Societies with high sodium intake show correspondingly high average blood pressures. The connection is not necessarily causal since many additional and uncontrollable factors are involved. Within a given society, blood pressure and sodium intake are usually weakly correlated at best. However, the uncertainties associated with estimating chronic sodium intake from single urine collections may obscure much stronger connections between salt and blood pressure. These epidemiological considerations have been discussed in a previous chapter, but further insight might be obtained from laboratory studies that have the needed control and precision.

Increases in salt intake, reduction of renal mass, and added mineralocorticoids are three procedures that can be used to raise blood pressure, but pressure often increases slowly and/or only slightly. In contrast, combinations of these interventions usually cause pressure to increase markedly and rapidly. In the rat, for instance, deoxycorticosterone acetate (DOCA) plus unilateral nephrectomy plus substitution of saline for drinking water is a popular and effective way to produce hypertension.

There is no guarantee that elevated dietary salt, subtotal nephrectomy and added mineralocorticoids individually involve the same pressor mechanisms. But, all three tend to increase the salt-and-water stores of the body and this appears to be a common and important factor.

Salt-and-water balance is a function of both intake and excretion. Sodium will accumulate if intake is excessive, excretion inadequate, or both. Sodium intake, particularly in the wild, is highly capricious; it therefore appears that renal excretion is under strong control and is primarily responsible for maintaining sodium homeostasis during unregulated intake.

INCREASED SODIUM INTAKE AND THE NORMAL ANIMAL

Increased arterial pressure accompanies increased dietary sodium intake in the normal animal. Rats are particularly susceptible to sodium excess (522),(643), but studies in chickens (574), dogs (965), primates (67),(148),(550), and humans (636),(685) have shown qualitatively similar results. Arterial pressure often increases slowly in these protocols and one year or more may elapse before genuine hypertension is observed. In addition, the term "high-salt diet" may refer to diets of up to 10 percent sodium chloride. This value is far in excess of human intake in all but a few isolated experimental situations. Nevertheless, arterial pressure correlates with sodium intake and the intake of large amounts of salt will lead to hypertension. The data of Meneely and colleagues is summarized below.

APPROXIMATE SYSTOLIC PRESSURE
AFTER 1 YEAR ON DIET (643)

Percent Salt in Diet	Systolic Pressure (mmHg)
.01	123
2.8	138
5.6	144
7.0	152
8.4	159
9.8	170

Dahl (201) and Meneely and Battarbee (642), among others, have enthusiastically reviewed the data relating increased blood pressure to increased salt intake.

LOSS OF RENAL MASS

As the total number of nephrons decreases, there are several important sequelae. The remaining renal mass tends to increase and this has been called compensatory hypertrophy. Blood flow and glomerular filtration rate in each nephron increase markedly as does each nephron's excretion of salt and water (29),(425). While whole-kidney values for flow and filtration are reduced, they are frequently still large enough to maintain normal salt and water excretion and the excretion of filtered metabolites such as urea and creatinine.

The upper limit of compensatory hypertrophy appears to be at about a doubling of flow and filtration in each nephron (426). When renal mass falls to about two-thirds of one kidney (or one third of the original total mass) compensatory hypertrophy is exhausted and increases in blood levels of filtered metabolites may become evident. Further reduction in renal mass leads to fatal uremia (103),(143),(357),(983), as first demonstrated over half a century ago in several species including the rabbit, cat, and dog. A protein-poor diet is beneficial when renal mass is low while a protein-rich diet worsens the uremia (12),(423). It appears that decreases in the nephron population first impair the excretion of filtered metabolites and the excretion of large amounts of sodium (27).

In 1932 Chanutin and Ferris (143) found that blood pressure might rise with subtotal nephrectomy to hypertensive levels. Pressure does not usually increase more than 5 or 10 mmHg in the dog when normal sodium intake is maintained, but considerably greater increases have sometimes been seen in the rat (143),(522),(523),(850),(1000).

HYPERTENSION FOLLOWING INCREASED SODIUM INTAKE AND DECREASED RENAL MASS

In the 1950's Koletsky and Goodsitt (522),(523) showed that increased sodium intake or decreased renal mass could separately produce hypertension in rats; but, the two together were a particularly potent combination. Their data is summarized below.

INCIDENCE OF HYPERTENSION IN KOLETSKY'S RATS

	Intact Kidneys	Unilateral Nephrectomy	Three-fourths Nephrectomy
Normal Salt	2.5%	16%	56%
1% Saline	66%	94%	100%

On a normal salt intake, unilateral nephrectomy increased arterial pressure and three-quarters nephrectomy increased it even farther. With both kidneys intact, increased sodium intake increased the incidence of hypertension relative to a fully intact animal on a normal salt intake. But, when increased salt intake was combined with unilateral nephrectomy the incidence rose to 98 percent. A 100 percent incidence of hypertension was seen when high salt intake was combined with three-quarter nephrectomy. Further, the onset of hypertension was much more rapid when the incidence of hypertension was high.

Langston *et al* (559) saw a similar response in dogs. Subtotal nephrectomy decreased glomerular filtration rate and increased blood urea nitrogen, indicating that the remnant kidney was just bordering on a filtration deficiency and that maximum sodium excretion was probably impaired. Superimposed administration of one-percent saline produced a rapidly developing hypertension which subsided when the saline was discontinued. Douglas *et al* (242) found evidence of blood and extracellular fluid volume expansion. Coleman and Guyton (168) observed an increase in cardiac output when salt loading was initiated. The cardiac output subsequently returned toward normal but blood pressure remained elevated because of increased total peripheral resistance. Right atrial pressure was elevated in these animals as evidence that volume expansion was forcing the increase in cardiac output. Manning *et al* (617) observed increased blood volume, right atrial pressure and mean circulatory filling pressure in similar studies. These data indicate that strong tendencies toward increased venous return develop with salt loading after subtotal nephrectomy. Recently, Liard (589) used micropheres to determine the distribution of vascular resistance several days after beginning salt-loading in subtotally nephrectomized animals. Cardiac output was elevated but at the same time most tissues were vasoconstricted. Skeletal muscle was not vasoconstricted and was accepting most of the excess flow. Subsequently, cardiac output and skeletal muscle flow returned to normal. Vasoconstriction is not homogeneous in this model; most tissues vasoconstrict faster than the whole-body resistance data has indicated, while skeletal muscle lags behind this response.

Plasma renin activity is decreased to low or undetectable levels when subtotal nephrectomy plus salt-loading is used to produce hypertension (524),(617).

In 1929, Verney (958) commented on the loss of functional renal mass and subsequent compensatory hypertrophy:

> "In the whole animal, therefore, it would not be surprising to find that when the second reserve of the kidney was exhaused and all the renal units were receiving the maximum stimulus which under the circumstances could be given them, and yet were unable to cope with the work thrust upon them, there should be a call for external aid in the form of a rise in the general blood pressure."

This quotation introduces a concept that brings sodium and the kidneys into the general scheme of blood pressure control: Excessive salt intake and reduced renal capacity create an extraordinary situation in which increased arterial pressure is needed to elevate salt-and-water excretion to a level at which sodium and volume homeostasis can be reestablished and maintained. The initially inadequate excretion and consequent fluid retention overdrive the circulation and provoke an autoregulatory vasoconstriction by the tissues (167),(391). The final result is increased peripheral resistance. Hence, initially high flow with normal resistance is replaced by high resistance and normal flow as hypertension continues.

This interpretation remains controversial (172) and part of the reason may be that unusual technical difficulties attend experimental verification. Firstly, hemodynamic transients have been given an important role in this explanation, but theoretically these transients would only be readily observed with very abrupt perturbations in volume homeostasis. More subtle pertubations with a gradually progressing hypertension would theoretically be associated with little change in volume, cardiac output, and other hemodynamic variables even though autoregulatory mechanisms were fully involved (172). A second problem is that transient disturbances soon disappear leaving little trace of what has happened. Thirdly, a powerful autoregulatory response would be more important than a weak one but more difficult to investigate experimentally because perturbations in flow would be dealt with rapidly and fully. Fourthly, many of the fundamental aspects of autoregulation are still not well understood. It is not clear, for instance, whether vasoconstriction with rising blood pressure should be considered metabolic or myogenic.

In 1976,Haddy and colleagues (397),(398) offered another explanation for the vasoconstriction that follows sodium retention. They argued that a hemodynamic explanation was unacceptable because changes in blood flow were not always observed during the onset of hypertension and because the autoregulatory response demonstrated by many tissues was much faster than the vasoconstriction described above. Sodium was postulated to have a direct effect on vascular smooth muscle leading to vasoconstriction. The idea: The sodium-potassium pump in smooth muscle is depressed during sodium retention; excessive salt and water will leak into the cells and vasoconstriction will result.

Specific connections between sodium retention and changes in the activity of sodium-potassium ATPase are not known. Extracellular sodium concentration usually remains relatively constant during the onset of salt-induced hypertension, but it has also been shown that salt-loading plus subtotal nephrectomy will produce hypertension during marked decreases in plasma sodium concentration (618). The quantity of sodium in the body and the extracellular fluid volume increase with salt-loading, but it has been difficult to postulate a functional connection between these variables and events within the cell membrane. Measurement of sodium-potassium ATPase activity in certain types of experimental hypertension has shown that this enzyme is often, but not always, depressed (398). Recently, Overbeck (726) has challenged Haddy's priority with regard to the idea that depressed sodium-potassium ATPase is the vasoconstrictor mechanism in salt-induced hypertension. The concept may not be developed enough at this time to quibble over.

Freidman and Freidman (326) have proposed a somewhat different scheme. They thought that leakage of sodium into vascular smooth muscle was excessive at the onset of hypertension. This increased leakage then was thought to stimulate, rather than depress, the sodium-potassium pump and to enhance protein synthesis. The result was postulated to be increased vascular smooth muscle tension, vasoconstriction and restructuring of the vessel wall. There is not enough data available at present to allow full evaluation of this idea.

ALDOSTERONISM

In 1953 though 1955, Simpson and colleagues extracted aldosterone from beef adrenal glands (867), determined its structure (868) and synthesized it (839). Deoxycorticosterone was already known to be a potent steroid and it would have been a likely suspect in instances of unusual sodium retention. But, Luetscher and Johnson (606) found another hormone in the urine of sodium-retaining patients. They tentatively, and correctly, identified it as aldosterone. In 1955, Conn (177),(178) fully described the consequences of a primary elevation in aldosterone formation and the benefits of surgical removal of the responsible tissue. Primary aldosteronism is also known as Conn's syndrome.

Aldosterone secreting tumors in humans provoke salt and water retention, excessive potassium excretion, hypokalemia, hypertension, and some evidence of eventual renal deterioration. Presumably the aldosterone excess acts primarily on the distal tubules of the kidney to enhance sodium reabsorption and potassium excretion. This leads to excess sodium stores (88) and hypertension while at the same time promoting hypokalemia. Blood pressure reduction can be achieved by sodium restriction, by use of diuretics, by pharmacological interventions that interfere with the synthesis or action of aldosterone (e.g., aminoglutethimide and spironolactone), and by surgical removal of the tumor.

Aldosterone has occasionally been used to produce hypertension in experimental animals. In 1957, Gross and colleagues (384) and Kumar *et al* (549) injected aldosterone and produced hypertension in the rat. Saline is often substituted for drinking water. Several recent reports describing aldosterone-induced hypertension in the rat (211),(530),(487) suggest that interest in this model is increasing once again. In these protocols, aldosterone appears to have roughly the same capacity as deoxycorticosterone in elevating blood pressure (401). Aldosterone infusions into dogs has produced mixed results. Both an increase (741) and no increase (598) in blood pressure have been reported; blood pressure may only rise when sodium intake is relatively high. Very little information is available concerning the mechanisms underlying pressure elevation with aldosterone administration, but it is widely assumed that sodium retention plays a critical role. A model substituting deoxycorticosterone acetate for aldosterone has been more widely studied.

DEOXYCORTICOSTERONE (DOCA) PLUS SALT

Deoxycorticosterone (DOCA), a potent mineralocorticoid, was synthesized by Steiger and Reichstein (892) in 1937. DOCA administration benefits those with adrenal insufficiency.

In 1940, Grollman and colleagues (380) first showed that DOCA will produce hypertension in the rat. Subsequently, this approach has been widely used in the rat and several other species. Blood pressure elevation is generally moderate to severe while a very severe, malignant form of hypertension sometimes develops (341). Plasma renin activity is suppressed to low or undetectable levels (645) and cannot be considered an important circulating hormone in this preparation. Cardiac output shows a tendency to increase at the onset of hypertension (181),(184). Increased extracellular fluid volume is often (181),(184), (341), but not always, observed. Late decreases in renal blood flow and glomerular filtration rate have been reported (327).

Rats have most often been used in DOCA plus salt

preparation and a standard procedure is to administer DOCA in a vehicle subcutaneously, to offer the animal isotonic or 1 percent saline as a substitute for drinking water and to remove one kidney. Blood pressure rapidly increases and remains elevated as long as the DOCA injection remains effective and saline is available to the animal. Blood pressure has been observed to both increase (402) and not increase (529) in animals with both kidneys intact. The arterial pressure increase with DOCA plus saline administration is about twice the increase when tap water is consumed *ad lib* (402).

DOCA without excess salt and without unilateral nephrectomy has been shown by Bohr and colleagues to cause hypertension in the pig (65),(651),(921). This hypertension is not associated with measureable volume expansion. It is often associated with severe hypokalemia. Hemodynamic measurements show small or no elevations in cardiac output at the onset of hypertension (651). Vascular reactivity to infused angiotensin and norepinephrine is increased (65). Sodium restriction corrects the hypokalemia but does not uniformly lower blood pressure (160). Thus, the pressure elevation appears to be a direct consequence of DOCA administration. Some effect of DOCA of vascular smooth muscle and/or intermediary neurogenic mechanisms might be involved.

Steroids, catecholamines, and the central nervous system

While steroid induced hypertension has been traditionally thought of in terms of salt and water excess, a variety of recent experiments have focused on central nervous system involvement. Takeda and Bunag (907) have observed increased sympathetic nerve activity in rats given DOCA plus salt. Reid and colleagues (789) and de Champlain *et al* (215) have observed increased plasma norepinephrine levels. Peripheral norepinephrine turnover is also increased (948),(347). The vasoconstriction produced by sympathetic nerve stimulation is greater than normal (255) but this cannot be ascribed to increased neurotransmitter release. Similarly Beilin and Wade (59) have observed a heightened blood pressure response to norepinephrine infusion in DOCA-salt hypertension. Heightened responsiveness might be a non-specific consequence of vessel wall hypertrophy (286),(287).

Six-hydroxydopamine injected into the cerebral ventricle prevents hypertension in this model over a period of several weeks (399),(546), (557),(789). However, ventricular 6-hydroxydopamine will not decrease pressure in established DOCA-salt hypertension (399),(546),(557). Peripheral sympathectomy with 6-hydroxydopamine has been shown to both prevent (217),(774) and not prevent (289) the onset of hypertension. Antiserum to nerve growth factor prevents the development of hypertension (38). In established DOCA-salt hypertension, peripheral sympathectomy has been observed to produce temporary (289) or partial (217) pressure decreases. Although the full range of effects of 6-hydroxydopamine are not known, it has been shown to effectively destroy the sympathetic nerve endings that it comes in contact with. (For a 1974 review of the biochemistry of 6-hydroxydopamine, see Kostrzewa and Jacobowitz (532)).

Fink *et al* (291) have shown that lesions in the central nervous system located at the anteroventral wall of the third ventricle prevent deoxycorticosterone-plus-salt hypertension in the rat. Thus, we have evidence of increased circulating catecholamines and evidence that the central components and possibly the perpheral components of the sympathetic nervous system play a permissive role in this model of hypertension.

The specific neural mechanisms involved in DOCA-salt hypertension have not been uncovered, and it may be that neural-renal factors enhance the antinatriuretic effects of DOCA. Katholi and colleagues (503) have shown that renal denervation prevents the development of DOCA-salt hypertension in rats. Renal vascular reactivity to infused norepinephrine and angiotensin has been shown to be increased (66), and neural influences on vascular smooth muscle in the kidney or smooth muscle in general might be important.

The critical interactions in the DOCA-salt model may involve salt excess rather than mineralocorticoid excess. Increased plasma catecholamines are normally associated with sodium deprivation (129),(607) presumably due to a reflex response to contracted body fluids and impending hypotension. But de Champlain, Carrierre and colleagues (139),(216) have advanced the idea that sympathetic nerve activity increases or becomes more effective with salt excess. Reid and colleagues (789) found increased plasma norepinephrine levels in rats becoming hypertensive with DOCA plus saline; but, they also found increased norepinephrine levels in rats that remained normotensive while receiving saline without DOCA. Both the ideas of increased catecholamines with sodium excess and increased catecholamines with sodium deprivation have received support from the recent study of Nicholls et al (693) who showed that plasma norepinephrine levels increase from normal values at high and low salt intakes. However, this observation is not supported by the work of Luft et al (607) and Weidmann and colleagues (979) who found progressively decreasing levels of plasma norepinephrine with increased sodium intake.

The possibility that salt might directly modify the sympathetic influence on renal function has been brought up in a preliminary report by Carriere (139). In response to renal nerve stimulation, renal vasoconstriction and renal vein catecholamines were greater in animals on a high salt diet, although background infusions of angiotensin complicated the protocol. Further support for salt-catecholamine-kidney interaction comes from the data of Cowley and Lohmeier (193) who produced hypertension in dogs by infusing norepinephrine directly into the renal artery at varying levels of sodium intake. In comparison to a low sodium intake, renal blood flow was lower and renal resistance was higher when the animals were on a high sodium intake even though the norepinephrine infusion rate had not been changed.

OTHER STEROIDS

A variety of other hormones have been shown to produce hypertension. Many of these models have not been studied in enough detail to provide insight into the general principles of blood pressure control.

Adrenocorticotropic hormone (ACTH) has been shown to stimulate adrenal steroid production and to produce hypertension in sheep (845),(846). But, the hypertension appears to be independent of both a direct pressor effect of ACTH (845), sodium retention (269), and known adrenal steroids (844),(846). It has been postulated then that ACTH stimulates adrenal production of a heretofore unfamiliar steroid which in turn produces hypertension by direct vascular effects. ACTH has also been shown to produce hypertension in the rat (314),(395). Metyrapone decreases cortisol secretion and stimulates ACTH release. It has been shown to produce a salt-sensitive hypertension in the dog (107),(720).

Glucocorticoids are often used therapeutically and

hypertension is occasionally observed. Glucocorticoid oversecretion, due to adrenal dysfunction or excessive ACTH stimulation, produces a wide spectrum of symptoms known as Cushing's syndrome; hypertension is often observed (765). Glucocorticoids (methylprednisolone) have been reported to increase blood pressure in the rat (536). Haack and colleagues (396) found that corticosterone produced a hypertension in the rat that was characterized by no change in salt and water balance but an increase in extracellular fluid and plasma volume. They concluded that a volume overload hypertension had been created by a shift of fluid from the intracellular to the extracellular compartments. In contrast, Hall *et al* (408) recently reported that glucocorticoids (methylprednisolone) had dramatic effects on glomerular filtration rate in the dog but little effect on blood pressure during a 10 day infusion.

In total, many different steroids will, at times, elevate blood pressure. Each steroid may involve unique pressor mechanisms, but it appears that hypertension most often develops when sodium intake exceeds the kidneys' excretory capacity. Increased arterial pressure would help to reestablish salt and water balance. The sympathetic nervous system may sometimes be involved but its exact role is not clear. There is usually a strong connection between salt and water retention and peripheral vasoconstriction but this connection appears to be too intricate to permit a simple explanation.

Sometimes, correlations between sodium retention and blood pressure do not develop. Take, for instance, the work of Nicholls *et al* (694). They found that fludrocortisone administration causes sodium retention and elevated blood pressure. However, these two variables were *negatively* rather than positively correlated. This should be taken as evidence against an important role for sodium retention in steroid hypertension. But there is another, rather speculative, explanation that gives sodium a causal role in the pressure increase while also suggesting how a negative correlation might develop. It may be that some subjects had a greater blood pressure sensitivity to sodium retention than others in this study. Sensitive subjects would reestablish sodium balance by way of a marked increase in pressure and this would require only minimal sodium retention. Less sensitive subjects would not develop as great a pressure increase and sodium balance would not be as readily reestablished. Balance would be achieved only after a greater amount of sodium had been retained and some factors other than increased pressure had finally improved excretion. Hence, blood pressure would increase because of sodium retention and at the same time a negative correlation between sodium and pressure would be seen since those with the least sodium retention would have the highest pressure and vice-versa.

CHAPTER 10

RENOPRIVAL HYPERTENSION

Hypertension appeared to result directly from bilateral nephrectomy in early studies, suggesting that nephrectomy terminated normal secretion of a depressor substance or normal metabolism of a pressor substance. But these protocols were often complicated by progressing uremia and lack of precise control of body fluids. More recently, chronic hemodialysis of anephric patients has shown that renoprival hypertension will not occur when precautions are taken to prevent overhydration. Blood pressure control in anephrics is linked to exchangeable sodium and extracellular fluid volume.

Although hypertension is not an invariable consequence of nephrectomy, a potentially important vasodepressor material has been demonstrated in renal tissue. Subcutaneous implants of homogenates or extracts of renal medulla will delay or prevent the onset of hypertension in experimental animals. Physiological importance has not yet been firmly established, however. Indirect evidence that a renal antihypertensive hormone may be active comes from instances in which changes in blood pressure involve the kidney but cannot be readily linked to changes in sodium excretion or the activity of the renin-angiotensin system. For instance, it has been shown that blood pressure will fall with repair of a renal artery stenosis ever when fluid loss is prevented. Such protocols demonstrate a short-term role in blood pressure control for unspecified renal antihypertensive factors, while leaving the question of a long-term role unsettled.

HYPERTENSION FOLLOWING BILATERAL NEPHRECTOMY

Renoprival hypertension is the hypertension that follows bilateral nephrectomy. One explanation is that nephrectomy ends renal secretion of a needed vasodilator substance. Another idea is that salt and water accumulate in the body after nephrectomy and that this accumulation has a hypertensive effect.

Early studies

The first observations of renoprival hypertension in anephric animals were complicated by the fact that long-term management of the resulting uremia was difficult or impossible. Both peritoneal dialysis and early applications of hemodialysis were attempted, but the results were less consistent in experimental animals than those obtained more recently in patients. In reviewing the animal studies it appears that normal hydration often preserved normotension while overhydration often led to hypertension (459),(527),(575),(722). Giovannetti and colleagues (349) found that bilaterally nephrectomized and dialized dogs remained normotensive when plasma and extracellular volumes were held constant; volume expansion over a week or so led to increased plasma and interstitial volume and hypertension. However, in several studies expanded fluid volume and increased cardiac output were not observed as hypertension developed (382),(675). These latter data imply that renoprival hypertension can sometimes have a humoral origin.

Early observations may have been complicated by changing body weights and the limited duration of the protocols. Over the long term, relatively small changes in fluid volume can produce large changes in arterial pressure in the anephric state; as a rule of thumb, arterial pressure will change 3 to 5 mmHg for every one percent change in body weight (166),(959).

Clinical studies

Patients with little excretory function but kidneys intact sometimes develop very severe hypertension even though fluid volumes are reduced using ultrafiltration and an artificial kidney. Plasma renin levels can rise to remarkably high levels in these instances and it often appears that the hyperreninemia is dominating blood pressure control (86),(806). This response is seen in some 10 or 20 percent of all dialysis patients (152),(959),(980).

The renin-angiotensin system is no longer a factor in the control of blood pressure when the kidneys are surgically removed. Most anephric patients show a striking pressure dependency on the salt and water stores of the body (100),(166),(644),(719),(817),(959). Ultrafiltration during hemodialysis lowers blood pressure; indiscriminate salt and water intake between dialyses raises blood pressure. Exceptions have been noted, however. Onesti and colleagues (718) have seen patients who do not show a blood pressure change with alterations in salt and water balance and the reason for this is not understood.

Blood pressure control in the anephric state

Patients undergoing chronic hemodialysis tend to become hypertensive. When hypertension develops immediately following nephrectomy, both expansion of body fluids and loss of renal vasodepressor hormones are plausible explanations. But when hypertension develops long after nephrectomy, the former explanation must be favored over the latter.

Increases in the body's salt and water stores lead to vasoconstriction. Elevated plasma sodium concentrations might be suspected of directly producing vasoconstriction, but acute increases in plasma sodium and osmolarity have actually been shown to cause vasodilation (727). Norman and colleagues (700) dialyzed anephric sheep and found that extracellular fluid volume had a pronounced effect on blood pressure while plasma sodium concentration or exchangeable sodium *per se* did not. Therefore, increases in blood pressure with overhydration seem to involve some connection between extracellular fluid volume and vascular smooth muscle tension.

Changes in extracellular fluid volume are shared by the plasma and interstitium (349). Ultrafiltration during hemodialysis has usually been observed to decrease body weight, plasma volume, cardiac output and arterial pressure (100),(362). Conversely, fluid retention between dialyses tends to increase cardiac output and arterial pressure.

Ledingham and Pelling (567) studied the hemodynamic response of anephric rats to overhydration. Arterial pressure increased with volume expansion and this was due to an increase in cardiac output. Changes in hematocrit or oxygen consumption did not appear to be responsible for the flow increase. Elevated flow was therefore judged to be a real overperfusion and it could have been capable of stimulating subsequent autoregulatory vasoconstriction. These animals were not dialyzed but were instead maintained on a low protein diet; therefore, observations were not possible beyond the first three or four days after nephrectomy. Coleman and colleagues (166) followed the transition from normotension to hypertension in a small group of anephric subjects. The first response to overhydration was an increase in cardiac output. Subsequently, increased peripheral resistance replaced increased cardiac output as the basis of the elevated arterial pressure. The time-course of hemodynamic events was considered by the authors to be consistent with an autoregulatory response.

Other studies indicate that the hemodynamic explanation is either incomplete or wrong. For instance, del Greco and colleagues (222) reported that cardiac output increased during hemodialysis in patients even though blood volume had been reduced. Such a response remains unexplained, but hemodialysis is a complicated clinical and physiological process and benefit to a failing heart or other unsuspected factors may have been involved. Kim and colleagues in Philadelphia have not favored a hemodynamic explanation since they seldom see the hemodynamic events described above (511).

Hatzinikolaou _et al_, (420) recently reported that acute manitol infusion in the absence of vasopressin expanded plasma volume but did not increase blood pressure in anephric rats. Hypertonic saline in the absence of vasopressin produced a comparable volume expansion but raised arterial pressure. Pressure increased even further in saline loaded anephric rats with normal pituitary function. The authors conclude that the pressure increase with volume expansion is partly due to vasopressin and partly due to some nonspecific effect of sodium and not at all due to hemodynamic factors.

The mechanisms involved in blood pressure control in the anephric state remain controversial, but several observations can be made. Firstly, hypertension can develop very readily in the absence of a functioning renin-angiotensin system. Secondly, arterial pressure tends to get out of control after bilateral nephrectomy, illustrating the importance of the kidneys in blood pressure control. Thirdly, nephrectomy eliminates the source of any vasodepressor materials of renal origin without necessarily producing hypertension. However, the loss of renal vasodepressors could contribute to the hypertensive tendencies mentioned above.

RENAL ANTIHYPERTENSIVE HORMONES

There are several ways in which humoral factors and the kidney could participate in the development of renoprival hypertension. One theory is that the kidney continually produces a renal vasodilator in quantities sufficient to cause normotension. A prediction of this theory is that secretion will terminate with bilateral nephrectomy and hypertension will invariably result. An alternative but similar concept is that a substance capable of producing hypertension is continually formed in the body and metabolized by the kidney. Here also nephrectomy will lead to hypertension. These theories have not been supported by the nearly universal observation that patients who are normotensive before bilateral nephrectomy remain normotensive following bilateral nephrectomy, if fluid volumes are properly maintained (100),(719), (959).

A different view is that a hormone having antihypertensive action is continually produced by the kidney and that renal disease, severe subtotal nephrectomy or bilateral nephrectomy reduce the circulating amount of this substance thereby predisposing the subject to hypertension. Neither the exact identity nor, in fact, the existence of this substance is settled, but prostaglandins and/or other substances of renal medullary origin having vasoactive properties might be involved. The kidney has been shown to be a rich source of vasoactive substances -- both pressor and depressor.

Renomedullary implants

In 1959, Muirhead and colleagues (679) reported that subcutaneous implantation of renal medulla would prevent hypertension from developing after bilateral nephrectomy. The antihypertensive properties of medulla and an associated lipid have been extensively studied over the ensuing two decades (669),(670). The lipid is either extracted from or contained in cell suspensions of fragmented renal medulla. Subcutaneous implantations of renal medulla, cultured renal interstitial cells, or extracted lipid have uniformly attenuated or prevented the onset of hypertension and have also lowered blood pressure in established hypertension. The following preparations have been studied: one-kidney Goldblatt (678),(673), two-kidney Goldblatt (619), angiotensin-plus-salt (677), renoprival (672),(674), partial nephrectomy-plus-salt (678), and Okamoto spontaneous hypertension (900). Even though arterial pressure was not fully and continually lowered in every instance, these studies show that there is a substance in the renal medulla that has potent hypotensive properties. It appears to act directly on the arterioles since changes in blood pressure occur without alterations in salt-and-water balance. Implantation protocols illustrate biochemical activity but not physiological importance.

With regard to the question of physiological importance, Susic and Kentera (899) have shown that experimental hypertension develops more readily when the renal medulla is missing. They used a special strain of rats in which some kidneys show congenital hydronephrosis. Salt-loading does not produce hypertension when animals have a fully functional kidney or when hydronephrosis is combined with a renomedullary implant; hypertension will develop with salt-loading when hydronephrosis is combined with a renocortical implant. Therefore, both intact medulla and implanted medulla demonstrate an antihypertensive function. This same approach was tried with one-kidney Goldblatt hypertension (901); the results show an antihypertensive effect for renomedullary implants but not for renal medulla that is distal to a Goldblatt clamp. The authors suggest that renal artery constriction interferes with the antihypertensive function of the medulla in situ. Using a different approach, Pitcock and colleagues (762) produced hypertension by partial nephrectomy and salt-loading. Renal papillae were taken from these hypertensive animals and implanted into other animals. The papillae had lost their ability to lower blood pressure.

In total, these studies show that a potent antihypertensive substance resides in the renal medulla. Physiological importance has been preliminarily indicated but has not yet been fully elucidated.

Manipulation of the ureters

Non-excretory renal function seems to modulate the pressure changes that occur with salt-loading. Floyer (302) and Muirhead and colleagues (676) have shown that salt-loading produces hypertension after bilateral nephrectomy and also when the kidneys are in place but the ureters are ligated. However, salt-loading does not change blood pressure when the ureters are implanted in the vena cava.

Lucas and Floyer (605) compared bilaterally nephrectomized rats to animals with a combination of unilateral nephrectomy and ureterocaval anastomosis. The bilaterally nephrectomized animals became hypertensive when salt-loaded; they showed a relatively uncompliant interstitium, a tendency for the extra fluid to stay within the circulation, and an increased venous pressure. In contrast, the animals with ureterocaval anastomosis did not become hypertensive; they showed a highly compliant interstitium and a tendency of this interstitium to absorb a large fraction of the overhydration. The concept being developed was that the normal animal does not develop hypertension when given a saline load because of rapid renal excretion and because renal mechanisms redistribute a large part of the load to the interstitium. Rapid excretion and redistribution would not occur in the anephric animal.

The data of Giovannetti and colleagues (349) is similar to that of Lucas and Floyer but not identical; bilateral nephrectomy plus saline led to hypertension while ureteral ligation plus saline did not. Bilaterally nephrectomized dogs showed increases in plasma and interstitial volume. Animals with ureteral ligation were properly volume expanded, but plasma volume remained constant while interstitial fluid volume increased markedly.

More recently, Liard (585) compared anephric dogs with those having ureterocaval anastomosis. Volume expansion produced a more pronounced increase in cardiac output in anephric animals, but this was more closely related to increases in cardiac function than to changes in the veins and interstitium. Manning (616) compared intact and anephric dogs and could not find evidence for changes in the function of the interstitium or changes in partition of fluid between the plasma and interstitium.

There is no single explanation for all observations involving salt-loading, nephrectomy, and manipulation of the ureter. The most uniform finding is that salt-loading produces hypertension after bilateral nephrectomy but does not produce hypertension when the ureter is implanted in the vena cava. Normotension with salt-loading is consistent with the idea that a renal depressor hormone is at work; but urine has been fed back into the circulatory system in these instances with uncertain, but probably not very physiological, consequences. Hypertension does not occur or occurs less readily when retained fluid accumulates in the interstitium rather than in the circulation. Except for the differences in excretory function, nephrectomized and intact dogs may be quite similar.

Acute renal transplantation

Indirect evidence for a pressor hormone of renal origin also comes from acute renal transplantation studies. Kolff and Page (526) and Muirhead et al (680) used dogs that were hypertensive after bilateral nephrectomy. Transplantation of normal kidneys to the hypertensive animals caused a rapid reduction in blood pressure that, at least in the latter study, wasn't associated with contraction of body fluids. Similar procedures have been used with animals having Grollman and DOCA-salt hypertension. Arterial pressure promptly fell with transplantation (355),(805) if the hypertension was not long-standing. Reduced pressure was caused by a decrease in cardiac output (805). Because of the rapidity of the response, a humoral explanation has been favored. But, inadvertent salt and water loss could have been a contributing factor. Presumably normal kidneys were perfused at initially high pressures in these protocols and volume contraction must be suspected unless there is compelling evidence to the contrary.

Renal antihypertensive hormones and functions have been investigated and discussed for several decades without full resolution of the details. Muirhead's lipid has been shown to be sufficiently potent, but its physiological importance is still in question. Plasma levels of other vasodepressor substances of renal origin, such as bradykinin and some of the prostoglandins, have not been satisfactorily linked to blood pressure changes. Most studies involving prostaglandins, for instance, have featured exogenous prostaglandins or powerful inhibitors rather than the endogenous prostaglandins themselves. Additional chemical and physiological data are needed.

NATRIURETIC HORMONE

Some confusion may result from the fact that several different and still unidentified hormones have been postulated to have a role in sodium balance and/or hypertension. Sodium excretion has been shown to be influenced by a variety of physical, humoral, and neural factors. But, changes in sodium excretion have been observed at times when the known excretory influences appear to be unchanged (224). These observations have inspired a persistent search for an additional hormone or hormones that could join the better known mechanisms in regulating sodium excretion. Such a hormone would oppose angiotensin, aldosterone and catecholamines in that elevated blood levels would promote natriuresis. It has accordingly been called "natriuretic hormone." An excellent review has been provided by Levinsky (577).

Most of the interest in natriuretic hormone has been related to control of sodium excretion and not to the mechanisms of hypertension. But, an absence of natriuretic hormone could theoretically lead to sodium retention and hypertension. The hormone being postulated by Haddy and colleagues (397),(398) is somewhat different. As discussed in a preceding chapter, Haddy is looking for a hormone that will induce vasoconstriction in response to positive sodium balance. As mentioned in this chapter, Muirhead has been investigating substances that appear to be directly vasoactive and, although they come from the kidney, they have not been directly tied to sodium excretion. In short, the putative natriuretic hormone relates to sodium excretion while Haddy and Muirhead have focused on the causes of vasoconstriction in hypertension.

CHAPTER 11

NEUROGENIC HYPERTENSION

Very high levels of circulating catecholamines, as seen in pheochromocytoma, will cause hypertension. But, less is known about more subtle functions within the central nervous system that can produce or prevent chronic hypertension. Attempts to develop a suitable animal model of neurogenic model remain controversial. Baroreceptor denervation was thought to produce hypertension by way of unchecked increases in sympathetic outflow. However, protocols utilizing continuous monitoring of blood pressure have indicated that lability, rather than the mean value of pressure, is increased in many instances. Lesions placed in the central nervous system have usually produced either a short-term fulminating hypertension or increased pressure lability only, but ablation of the nucleus of the tractus solitaris has now been shown to produce sustained increases in blood pressure. Recent studies have also indicated that there are permissive neural factors; normal nervous function is needed for the production of several types of experimental hypertension. In some instances, chronic hypertension has been produced using imposed stresses that presumably increase sympathetic activity.

CATECHOLAMINES AND HYPERTENSION

Many clinicians and investigators feel that the autonomic nervous system plays a very important role in the etiology of essential hypertension. This conclusion is indirectly supported by the observation that vasoconstriction invariably accompanies high blood pressure and by the known potency of catecholamines in producing vasoconstriction. It has proved difficult, however, to support this contention with direct evidence. Attempts to develop a suitable animal model have had mixed success.

A catecholamine producing tumor, called a pheochromocytoma, can raise plasma norepinephrine and epinephrine concentrations to very high levels in humans (600) and a severe hypertension results, as recently reviewed by Manger and Gifford (615). This hypertension is treated by pharmacological agents that block the effect of catecholamines on vascular smooth muscle (such as phenoxybenzamine and phentolamine) and the hypertension is usually cured by surgical excision of the tumor. Transplanted pheochromocytoma tumor has also been shown to produce hypertension in rats (972). Attempts to produce chronic hypertension by catecholamine infusion have led to mixed results; these will be reviewed in a following chapter.

Plasma catecholamines have been measured in human essential hypertension and in many forms of experimental hypertension. Increased levels have sometimes been observed, but these increases have not been large enough to allow firm conclusions. The case of human hypertension will be reviewed in more detail in a later chapter.

THE BLOOD PRESSURE RESPONSE TO BARORECEPTOR DENERVATION

Blood pressure rises when the afferent arm of the baroreceptor reflex is severed. Nerves leaving the carotid sinus and aortic arch region are sectioned using surgical procedures that account for anatomical variations among the rat (538), rabbit (101) and dog (440),(474),(475),(703). The baroreceptors in the chest appear to be more important than those in the neck since carotid sinus denervation alone does not elevate blood pressure (476) while denervation at the aortic arch produces mild hypertension (292),(477).

Both the acute and persistent pressure increases are characterized by increased pressure lability, increased catecholamines (10) and varied vasoconstriction (8),(89),(279),(541). These data indicate that the baroreceptor reflexes constantly stabilize and restrain blood pressure; loss of restraint leads to a blood pressure elevation that is commonly called neurogenic hypertension. Probably a better name would be "baroreceptor-denervation hypertension" since there are several different types of "neurogenic" hypertension.

Cowley *et al* (192) measured blood pressure continuously in debuffered dogs and found out that aortic pressure showed an increased lability but a normal mean pressure. That is, blood pressure was very poorly controlled over the short-term; but, for every upward excursion from the norm there was eventually a comparable downward excursion and the 24-hour mathematical average for blood pressure remained normal. Norman and Coleman (699) have reported that debuffered rats show a normal blood pressure when left unattended and an elevated pressure when handled. Cardiovascular restructuring usually accompanies persistent hypertension. However, Jones and Hallback (489) did not find any evidence of restructuring in debuffered rats that appeared to be hypertensive. It is clear that arterial pressure is much lower in the debuffered animal when environmental stimuli are at a minimum (192),(497),(699). It may be that the hypotensive and hypertensive episodes are just about offsetting over an extended period leaving the long-term mean arterial pressure at a normal level. These results suggest that the baroreceptors have a very important role in the short-term control of blood pressure but much less of a role in long-term control.

Scher presents another side of the story (834). He argues that an increase in mean arterial pressure would not be expected if debuffering is incomplete. As an example, Guyton and colleagues (390) have shown that arterial pressure remains relatively stable with partial surgical denervation but that gross instability occurs after all of the afferent nerves are cut; this is independent of the denervation sequence. The usual tests, such as heart rate decrease with pressor injections of phenylephrine, may not be sensitive enough to characterize complete denervation. But if this argument is to stand, its proponents must explain the differential mechanisms by which increased pressure lability accompanies almost all surgical denervations while real increases in mean pressure remain more elusive. If debuffering leads directly to hypertension, increases in mean pressure and pressure lability should be roughly proportional.

LESIONS IN THE CENTRAL NERVOUS SYSTEM

Lesions in the brain have been known to produce hypertension. There are isolated clinical reports of long-standing hypertension in human beings that upon subsequent autopsy show clear signs of central nervous system involvement. Incidental observations such as these have not added much to our understanding. The development of suitable animal models has shown that lesions in the brain can both cause and prevent hypertension.

Lesions that elevate blood pressure

The nucleus of the tractus solitarus (NTS) is located in the brainstem. It appears to be an intermediary between baroreceptor afferents and the vasomotor and vagal centers. Nerves that use norepinephrine as a neurotransmitter both originate and terminate there (142).

Doba and Reis (236),(237) abolished the baroreceptor reflexes and produced large elevations in arterial pressure by bilateral ablation of the nuclei of the tractus solitaris. The pressure rise was extremely rapid and this hypertension was therefore characterized as "fulminating." Death results in 12 hours or so after ablation. The pressure increase and its sequelae can be prevented by phentolamine, peripheral sympathetomy and adrenalectomy, or regional sympathetomy produced by injecting 6-hydroxydopamine into the cisterna magna. Hence, this particular lesion in the rat causes an intense neurogenic vasoconstriction (884) but the model cannot be considered a strict neuogenic model of hypertension if the chronic element is missing.

More recent studies have shown that lesions in and around the nucleus of the tractus solitaris can cause very specific changes in baroreceptor function that may include long-standing increases in arterial pressure. A2 neurons somehow relate the nucleus of the tractus solitaris to vagal control of heart rate. Selective A2 destruction results in a loss of the heart rate response to baroreceptor stimulation while the peripheral sympathetic component is maintained (914). The lability of blood pressure is increased but not the mean level. A comparable response has been produced by local injection of 6-hydroxydopamine into the NTS (885) although there is no guarantee that the same neural mechanisms are involved. Zandbert et al (1009) confirmed NTS lesions produced acute increases in blood pressure with elevated plasma renin and epinephrine levels. But more importantly, they demonstrated that hypertension was sustained for up to six weeks. Nathan and Reis (689) showed that similar lesions in the cat will abolish the baroreceptor reflex and produce a sustained hypertension that is typified by both increased pressure lability and an elevation in the mean level of pressure. Most recently, destruction of the NTS has been shown to produce sustained hypertension in the dog (137),(562). These data in total show that destruction of the nucleus of the tractus solitaris interrupts the baroreceptor reflex and rapidly increases arterial pressure. A sustained hypertension evolves that is characterized by peripheral vasoconstriction of neural origin. However, this model cannot be considered to be identical to that produced by surgical interruption of the baroreceptor afferent nerves at this time.

Lesions that prevent hypertension

Injection of 6-hydroxydopamine into the cerebral ventricles has been shown to depress noradrenergic function and to prevent the onset of several types of experimental hypertension. It appears that normal noradrenergic function in the central nervous system is a prerequisite for the development of hypertension in general. These studies are referred to in the chapters addressed to specific types of experimental hypertension.

Lesions in the preoptic region of the anterior hypothalamus have also been shown to prevent blood pressure increases. Brody and colleagues (111),(112) have investigated the consequences of destroying the periventricular tissue of the anterior and lateral regions of the third ventricle (AV3V) in the rat. Thirst, the control of blood osmolarity, renal excretion, the response to injected angiotensin, and the blood pressure response to hypertensive stimuli are all altered by AV3V lesions. Figure-of-eight ligature (Grollman) plus contralateral nephrectomy hypertension is prevented (124), as is DOCA-salt hypertension (291). Buggy *et al* (123) have shown that AV3V lesions will reduce arterial pressure in established Grollman and two-kidney Goldblatt hypertension. Curiously, the development of Okamoto hypertension is not altered by AV3V lesions (123),(359) and this remains unexplained. However, the data in total suggest that the integrity of this region of the anterior hypothalamus is required for the development of hypertension in general. Considering the "renal" nature of the experimental models investigated, it is likely that AV3V lesions produce striking changes in the function of the kidneys.

Brody *et al* (112) favor a causal role for the AV3V region in the development of hypertension rather than just a permissive role, but this contention does not have strong experimental support at the present time.

STRESS AND HYPERTENSION

The unusual prevalence of essential hypertension in blacks has fostered the notion that a stressful environment, such as living in a ghetto, produces or enhances hypertension (416). Also, certain professions (e.g., air traffic controller) might provide enough inherent stress to cause hypertension. The normal response to stress includes tachycardia, increased cardiac output, vasodilation (377),(441) and an increase in muscle blood flow (108). However, some normotensive (441) and many hypertensive (109),(428),(691),(828),(855) subjects show an atypical response that includes abnormally large blood pressure elevations and vasoconstriction rather than vasodilation.

The underlying idea is that the stress reaction evolved in man as a nervous response that readied the body for strenuous physical activity; in modern society physical activity seldom accompanies stress and serious cardiovascular consequences may result, particularly in predisposed individuals. It has also been postulated that a series of acute blood pressure elevations might cause some permanent changes in the vasculature, and particularly the renal vasculature, leading to sustained hypertension (114),(427). Folkow (303),(304) has expanded this idea with the concept that it takes little or no additional stimulation to maintain vasoconstriction once hypertension has continued long enough to cause the blood vessel walls to hypertrophy. Confirmation in the clinical setting has been a difficult undertaking and, consequently, there have been many attempts to develop an animal model in which hypertension follows environmental stress. The selection of meaningful stresses and relevance to the human condition remain unsettled.

It has been shown that imposed stresses elevate arterial pressure in a variety of animal models, although blood pressure elevations have sometimes been modest and/or short-lived. Herd *et al* (436) produced blood pressure and heart rate increases in primates by repetitive electrical shocks; pressure rose slowly, but sustained hypertension was eventually demonstrated in 4 of 6 animals studied. Loud noises, flashing lights, vibrations and other stimuli have been used to elevate pressure in rats (270),(463),(752). Henry and colleagues (434),(435),(953) have produced a most convincing demonstration of the connection between environmental stress and hypertension. In a specially designed housing device, rats maturing in overcrowded conditions had higher blood pressures than rats maturing in quarters where overcrowding was not present.

It is still not completely clear under what conditions persistent hypertension results from reasonable stresses. Some insight may come from the data of Friedman and Iwai (322). They showed that the Dahl "salt-sensitive" substrain of spontaneously hypertensive rat will become hypertensive with stress while the "salt-resistant" substrain will not. Similarly, Rothlin et al (808) were not able to produce hypertension in albino laboratory rats using loud noises. The same procedures did produce hypertension, however, in offspring produced by cross-breeding the laboratory rats with wild Norway rats. The implication is that stress will more readily lead to hypertension in those subjects that have a particular, predisposing genetic background (335).

The converse might also hold; that is, relaxation, a pleasant environment, transcendental meditation, or reassuring encounters might lower blood pressure in some subjects. To date, only small and usually acute decreases in blood pressure have been reported in clinical studies (64),(745). Detailed reviews of psychotherapy have been provided by Steptoe (894) and Shapiro and colleagues (857).

A CONNECTION BETWEEN BLOOD PRESSURE, THE NERVOUS SYSTEM AND THE KIDNEYS

Increased sympathetic activity could increase arterial pressure by direct vasoconstriction, increased myocardial contractility (587), (588), venous effects or renal mechanisms.

The kidneys have a rich sympathetic innervation (48). Early studies showed that stimulation of the renal sympathetic nerves would decrease renal blood flow, glomerular filtration rate and sodium and water excretion (458). Recently DiBona and associates (225),(878) have reported that low-level nerve stimulation can produce an antinatriuresis and antidiuresis without concomitant decreases in flow and filtration. They postulate that a direct effect of the autonomic nerves on tubular reabsorption provides a connection between nervous outflow and renal excretion without involving hemodynamic intermediates. There is some anatomical evidence in support of their argument (49).

A neurogenic model of hypertension resulting from neurally mediated decreases in renal function would probably have many features in common with the many other models of hypertension that depend on manipulation of the kidneys. In the late 1940's, Kottke and Kubicek (533),(544) demonstrated that splanchnic or renal nerve stimulation produced marked hypertension in dogs. When the electrical stimulation was discontinued, the blood pressure rapidly fell back to normotensive levels. We have not been able to reproduce this (unpublished observation, Drs. Roger Norman and Thomas Coleman).

A preliminary report by Kline and colleagues (514) indicates that renal denervation prevents baroreptor-denervation hypertension. It may be that renal denervation interferes with sodium conservation. The tendency for pressure to vaccilate upwards after debuffering would be offset by a volume contracted state. They (517) have also reported that inhibition of converting enzyme prevents debuffering hypertension; this data suggests that the pressor and/or antinatriuretic effects of angiotensin are important in this model.

CHAPTER 12

HYPERTENSION DUE TO INFUSED VASOCONTRICTOR AGENTS

Acute infusions have been used to demonstrate the vasoconstrictor potency of angiotensin II, norepinephrine, and vasopressin (antidiuretic hormone). It follows that chronic administration might produce sustained hypertension, but this has not been the case in each instance. Continuous infusion of angiotensin, even at relatively low rates, produces sustained hypertension. Continuous infusion of even maximal amounts of norepinephrine in dogs produces at best a moderate sustained increase in pressure; blood pressure in humans may be more sensitive to catecholamine producing tumors. Vasopressin infusion initially elevates arterial pressure but the response wains.

The pressor effects of angiotensin have been studied in detail. Intrarenal infusions are just as effective as intravenous infusions in elevating blood pressure, demonstrating an antinatriuretic component to the hypertensive response. Infusion into the vertebral arteries also produces hypertension. These data suggest that the total response to angiotensin infusion has three components : direct vasoconstriction, augmentation of the vasoconstriction by neural factors, and an antinatriuretic effect that maintains fluid volumes in the face of high renal perfusion pressure or even adds to the hypertension via fluid retention.

ANGIOTENSIN INFUSION

In the 1960's, it was first shown that chronic angiotensin infusion would produce hypertension in rabbit (113),(228),(230),(1008), and dog (634),(713), and man (16). The hypertension is due to vasoconstriction; cardiac output tends to be a little low, particularly at the beginning of the infusion, or normal (713),(1001). Pressure rises gradually when relatively small amounts of angiotensin are used. After a week or so, the pressure increment may be more than twice the initial rise.

Possible reasons for the delayed pressure increase during angiotensin infusion have been widely investigated. One possibility is that the responsiveness of the blood vessels to angiotensin increases with prolonged infusion. This idea is not supported by the data of Bean and colleagues (57), however. They saw no changes in vascular responsiveness while hypertension was developing during two weeks of low-level infusion. Another possibility is that the baroreceptors oppose the initial increase in pressure but, because of adaptation, offer little long-term hindrance. This idea is supported by the data of Cowley and DeClue (189). They showed that low levels of angiotensin infusion into baroreceptor-denervated dogs resulted in a rapid increase in arterial pressure. Blood pressure rose more slowly when the same procedures were used with intact dogs.

The renal effects of angiotensin may be important. Sodium retention has been observed during angiotensin infusion, although the amount is usually not very large (16),(405),(598),(707),(1001). Mean circulatory filling pressure, an estimate of the net hemodynamic effect of changes in venous compliance and blood volume, has been reported to be increased during long-term intravenous infusions (1001). This indicates that a relative overhydration has developed that could either be due to angiotensin-mediated volume expansion or a change in the function of the veins. It has also been shown that pressure increases are greater for a specific angiotensin infusion rate when the animal is on a high-salt diet (194),(219). This might be due to a direct effect of sodium on the vasculature, but it is more likely the result of interaction between the antinatriuretic effect of angiotensin and the salt load.

Using a more direct approach, Lohmeier and Cowley (597) showed that hypertension could be produced by infusing angiotensin directly into the renal artery. Renal blood flow, glomerular filtration rate and sodium excretion decreased when the infusion was initiated. Sodium was retained. Plasma renin activity fell to very low levels. These changes were reversed when the infusion was terminated. It may be that a fraction of the infused angiotensin leaves the kidney by way of the renal veins, recirculates, and causes some direct arterial constriction. If recirculation is not significant, two conclusions seem warranted. 1) The antinatriuretic and/or other renal effects of angiotensin *per se* are powerful enough to produce hypertension. 2) During intravenous angiotensin infusions, the renal effects of angiotensin seem to prevent pressure-induced volume contraction and they may, in fact, contribute to the gradual blood pressure increase.

When Dickinson and Lawrence (228) first demonstrated that pressure slowly rises with chronic low-level angiotensin infusion, thay speculated that the gradual increase might be due to some effect of angiotensin on the brain resulting in sympathetic vasoconstriction. It was subsequently shown that angiotensin will increase blood pressure when infused into the vertebral artery (276),(1007),(1008). Fukiyama and colleagues (331) then showed that chronic vertebral infusion causes sustained, although mild, blood pressure increases. Angiotensin might elicit this response by constricting the cerebral circulation, but areas have been identified where angiotensin can enter the brain without hindrance from the blood-brain barrier (277). Two questions remain unanswered. Do blood angiotensin levels increase enough during intravenous infusion to elicit a central nervous system response? Does the response have some characteristic that would lead to a gradual pressure increase?

Angiotensin is a potent vasoconstrictor in the absence of a functional nervous system (190) and has antinatriuretic effects in the denervated kidney (978). Hence, intravenous infusion may cause a combination of direct vasoconstriction, inhibition of salt and water excretion, and increased autonomic outflow. Although the quantitative importance of each of these components is not certain, it's likely that angiotensin directly vasoconstricts the arterioles in most angiotensin infusion protocols.

NOREPINEPHRINE INFUSION

Norepinephrine secreting tumors have been shown to produce hypertension in humans (615) and this same tumor tissue when transplanted to the rat also causes hypertension (972).

The pressure response during long-term norepinephrine infusion has been inconsistent. Blacket and colleagues (94) saw toxic manifestations rather than sustained hypertension with intravenous infusion into rabbits. In contrast, Dickinson and de Swiet (218),(227) stayed below toxic levels and produced a moderate, gradually-developing hypertension. Success depended on continually increasing the infusion rate, however. Laks and colleagues (340),(556) found that intravenous infusion of rather large amounts of norepinephrine into dogs led to an increase in cardiac output rather than an increase in arterial pressure.

Intrarenal norepinephrine infusion through catheters placed in the renal artery has been shown to produce hypertension (193),(502) although the pressure elevations observed are not as great as those seen in some other experimental models. The cause of the increased pressure is not certain. Total peripheral resistance is elevated and cardiac output is depressed (502). Sodium retention occurs on the first day of infusion (502), but the depressed cardiac output is evidence against the idea that this is a salt-induced hypertension. Blood flow through the kidney is decreased. Marked increases in plasma renin activity at the beginning of infusion (502) are followed by lesser but sustained increases (193), (502). Vasoconstriction may be of neural origin since phentolamine rapidly drops blood pressure back to normal. Some of the infused norepinephrine leaves the kidney by way of the renal veins and enters the systemic circulation (502); the pressor effect of this circulating norepinephrine does not appear to be large, however.

Although quantitative comparison is difficult, intrarenal norepinephrine infusion may be superior to intravenous infusion in producing long-term elevations in arterial pressure. If so, renal factors are a very important part of catecholamine-induced hypertension.

VASOPRESSIN OR ANTIDIURETIC HORMONE INFUSION

In 1895, Oliver and Schafer (711) demonstrated that the pituitary contained a vasopressor substance. In the 1950's, DuVigneaud and colleagues determined the structure (247) of the peptide vasopressin and synthesized it (246). Vasopressin is normally thought of as antidiuretic hormone, a substance that corrects osmotic imbalances by adjusting the amount of water in the body to exactly match the amount of available sodium. The repercussions of a loss of antidiuretic hormone have been studied in rats with hereditary diabetes insipidus (946),(947) -- the Brattleboro strain. Water turnover is extremely high. Disturbances in the amount and osmolarity of extracellular fluid have been observed (325), but abnormal arterial pressures have not been seen (200), (235),(400).

Acute vasopressin infusions have shown that this hormone is a potent vasoconstrictor. Blood pressure rises, cardiac output decreases, blood flow is redistributed, and salt and water excretion is altered. There is also good evidence that endogenous antidiuretic hormone can increase in the blood to vasopressor levels (195),(563),(775),(801). Continuous vasopressin infusion into dogs has been shown to produce mild increases in blood pressure that are not sustained (880). Hence, vasopressin seems to be more active in short-term than in long-term control of blood pressure.

Recent, but indirect, evidence in the support of the idea that vasopressin has a long-term role in control of blood pressure comes from the observation that rats with hereditary diabetes insipidus will not develop DOCA-salt hypertension (200) while comparable rats with normal pituitary function will. Dlouha *et al* (235) observed a similar resistance to the development of hypertension, but mild pressure increases were observed in young animals that were uninephrectomized and given saline to drink. Several studies from 3 or 4 decades ago (104),(708),(736) showed that hypophysectomy generally lowered blood pressure in normotensive and hypertensive animals, but the hypotensive effect seemed to be closely connected to loss of proper adrenal function.

Plasma vasopressin concentration has been shown to be moderately elevated in several forms of hypertension (199),(655),(657), (658). While the blood levels seen do not indicate that vasopressin is having a major pressor role (728), vasopressin blockade with analog (200) or antibody (655),(657),(658) has been observed to produce striking decreases in blood pressure. The reason for this disparity between vasopressin levels and apparent pressor effects is not known. The infusion data cited above suggests that the pressure decrease with blockade might turn out to be only temporary; the blood pressure response to chronic blockade has not been reported.

CHAPTER 13

GENETIC OR SPONTANEOUS HYPERTENSION IN ANIMALS

Studies of human essential hypertension have shown that there is a strong genetic component to this disease, as reviewed in a previous chapter. Children whose parents have essential hypertension have a much greater than normal chance of having essential hypertension themselves as they reach adulthood. But, this statistical connection does not show us what gene or genes are involved or how the genetic information is conveyed to the physiological processes that ultimately influence blood pressure.

The physiology of genetic hypertension has been investigated using animals that predicably develop hypertension under genetic influence. These special strains have been created by breeding pairs of animals with unusually high blood pressures and then by repeatedly inbreeding the strain until hypertension is observed in all or most of the offspring. Various species have been used, with the rat receiving the most attention. Practical considerations in developing special hypertensive strains include fertility, period of gestation, and litter sizes. The rat has apparently been very suitable in this regard.

Although there are a variety of strains and substrains of animals that become hypertensive without further intervention, there is no guarantee that the physiological mechanisms involved are the same in each instance. In fact, this would be highly unlikely; in the absence of evidence to the contrary,we must assume that any number of mechanisms are involved. For instance, an inborn adrenal defect might be centered in the adrenal cortex. Hypertension would result from excessive aldosterone secretion. Another adrenal defect might involve the adrenal medulla and produce hypertension by excessive catecholamine secretion. In both instances the adrenal gland would have primary involvement and the result would be high blood pressure, but the physiological details would be vastly different.

A further uncertainty comes from the possibility that

genetic drift may be occurring. For instance, the Okamoto strain of spontaneously hypertensive rats has been widely disseminated and many isolated colonies are now in existence. We have no guarantee that the mechanisms increasing blood pressure are identical in widely separated colonies since, in many instances, numerous generations have passed since the colony was splintered from the parent strain. Inconsistencies in observations have occurred and genetic drift is one possible explanation.

Two uses can be made of spontaneously hypertensive animals: one is to study the genetic transmission of high blood pressure using breeding and cross-breeding protocols and the second is to use the animals in experiments that might reveal the physiological mechanisms underlying the blood pressure increase. Cross-breeding experiments require two strains that have been specifically bred to emphasize and de-emphasize a particular trait. This criterea has not often been met in blood pressure research. One exception is the Dahl strain of spontaneously hypertensive rat which has in fact two substrains suitable for cross-breeding. Many other strains are less suitable and the appropriateness of control animals used in many experiments has been the source of persistent controversy. In particular, the Okamoto strain was derived from Wistar laboratory rats but for some time there was no control strain comparably inbred for low blood pressure. Now a Kyoto Wistar strain has been developed ond offered as a suitable control.

Physiological experimentation with spontaneously hypertensive animals has in some instances not involved hypothesis formulation and testing but instead has involved looking for measurable differences between hypertensive and normotensive groups. This approach has proved to be rather frustrating since so few differences, in addition to the marked blood pressure difference, have been observed. Further, obvious differences may be entirely secondary to the blood pressure increase. There are many additional experiments, however, that are scientifically valid and illuminating.

The spontaneously hypertensive animal, and rat in particular, has at times been heralded as a superb experimental analog of essential hypertension. This has been criticized in light of the fact that essential hypertensives show a wide variety of hemodynamic, humoral, and nervous traits while strains of spontaneously hypertensive animals tend to highly uniform. This discussion can be profitably continued when more is known about the mechanisms underlying essential hypertension and genetic hypertension. To date, however, both subjects with essential hypertension and these specially prepared strains of animals have been remarkably zealous in not revealing the mechanisms underlying the blood pressure increase.

Four strains of spontaneously hypertensive rats are described in the following chapters. They are:

1. the Okamoto strain from Japan.
2. the Dahl substrains of salt-sensitve and salt-resistant rats from Brookhaven National Laboratory, Long Island, New York.
3. the New Zealand genetically hypertensive rat.
4. the Milan or Bianchi hypertensive rat from Italy.

Spontaneous hypertension in these four strains has recently been carefully reviewed by Folkow and Hallback (309). The possible importance of renal factors in these animals has also been discussed (171).

CHAPTER 14

GENETIC HYPERTENSION: THE OKAMOTO STRAIN OF RATS

The Okamoto strain of spontaneously hypertensive rats was created in Japan in the early 1960's and since that time it has become the most widely studied experimental model in hypertension research. A resemblance to human essential hypertension has been noted in that blood pressure increases gradually with time in both the Okamoto rat and the subject with essential hypertension, and the cause of the pressure increase remains unknown in both cases. Of the many experimental observations available for analysis, the following three may be the most relevant. Sympathetic nervous activity is significantly increased in these rats. Renal denervation has been shown to prevent hypertension as long as the denervation remains effective. When the kidneys are cross-transplanted between hypertensive animals and normotensive controls, the ultimate level of pressure is determined by the donor kidney rather than the recipient animal.

THE ORIGIN OF THE OKAMOTO RAT

This strain was developed by Professor Kozo Okamoto (710) at Kyoto University beginning in the early 1960's. The Okamoto rat quickly became very popular and widely disseminated. An excellent summary of the early investigations into the cause of hypertension in this strain was published in 1972 (709).

The popularity of the Okamoto rat probably depends in part upon the large and very predictable increase in blood pressure that occurs as the animals mature. However, most investigations to date have shed little light on the mechanisms controlling arterial pressure in this strain. Many investigators currently feel that the central nervous system and increased autonomic outflow play an important role in the hypertension of the Okamoto spontaneously hypertensive rat.

HEMODYNAMICS

Hemodynamic data from Okamoto rats are divided between observations of increased cardiac output and observations of normal cardiac output. Much of the data has come from anesthetized, thoracotomized animals and such surgical preparation could create or obscure differences in flow. Iriuchijima and colleagues (473),(704) compared Okamoto hypertensive rats of up to one year of age to normotensive controls and found no differences in cardiac output. Prewitt and Dowell (769) found no differences. In contrast, Pfeffer and Frohlich (755) and others (6),(906) have observed increased cardiac output in Okamoto rats, particularly in young animals (881). Propranolol will lower cardiac output and oxygen consumption (996) but will not prevent the development of hypertension in this strain (756).

These data indicate that cardiac output is sometimes, but not always, elevated in Okamoto hypertension. Smith and Hutchins (881) have suggested that elevated cardiac output in young animals might trigger autoregulatory vasoconstriction. But, increased oxygen consumption (906),(996) has been seen in Okamoto rats and elevated flows might therefore represent a normal hemodynamic response to altered metabolic conditions. Indirect evidence in support of autoregulatory vasoconstriction comes from an entirely different experimental approach. Folkow and colleagues (306),(982) used aortic ligation to reduce arterial pressure only in the hindquarters of Okamoto rats. The resistance at maximum dilation and vascular responsiveness in the hindquarters decreased with time to values that could be considered normal for the new prevailing blood pressure. These data show that some aspects of the vasoconstriction in Okamoto rats are autonomous and independent of whole-body humoral and neural influences.

Determinations of blood volume and exchangeable sodium have shown values that are in general normal (43),(824),(939) or slightly depressed (797),(840). Its not likely that normal to high cardiac outputs could be maintained with normal to low blood volumes unless additional hemodynamic factors were involved. And furthermore, the very high arterial blood pressure seen in these animals places an unusual load on the left heart that can depress cardiac function (412),(753). Several studies have found decreased venous compliance in Okamoto rats (366),(824), (863) and this might help to compensate for contracted fluid volumes and increased cardiac afterload.

Samar and Coleman (824) observed normal blood volume but decreased venous compliance in Okamoto rats. Mean circulatory filling pressure, an indicator of the total hemodynamic value of blood volume and vascular compliance combined, was measured and was found to be elevated 18%. These animals, therefore, showed normal blood volume but functional overhydration. The increased mean circulatory filling pressure might have a role in the genesis of the hypertension or, at least, it would help to maintain cardiac output in the face of increased cardiac afterload. In support of this latter idea, Noresson and colleagues (698) found that left atrial pressure was elevated in Okamoto rats. While the cause of decreased venous compliance in these animals is not known, it will be noted in a later chapter that many patients with essential hypertension show very similar hemodynamic characteristics.

The microcirculation

Increased resting arteriolar tone is thought to supply the vasoconstriction in hypertension in general, although in some instances this is more assumption than fact. Inspection of Poiseuille's equation for the determinants of resistance to flow indicates that increased blood viscosity, increased resistance vessel length, or decreased numbers of resistance vessels are theoretically just as suitable sources of increased resistance as is arteriolar vasoconstriction. The spontaneously hypertensive rat is particularly interesting because it "grows up" with its hypertension. Growth of a lesser number of vessels, called vessel rarefaction, might replace or supplement arteriolar constriction as the source of increased vascular resistance. In the opposite direction, hypotension (180) has been clearly shown to stimulate the growth of blood vessels.

Special microscopic techniques have been used to visualize and measure small blood vessels in the Okamoto rat. Small arteries may be of normal length (467) or shortened (433). The size of the lumen in these vessels is slightly increased (433),(467). One of the most striking observations has been that the number of small arteries is about one-half of that seen in normotensive Wistar Kyoto control rats (433),(467). Vascular permeability and lymph flow are increased (438).

Bohlen *et al* (96) and others (439) have measured pressures in the cremaster muscle and mesentery. Pressures are elevated on both the arterial and venous sides. But, a particularly large pressure drop from the large arteries to capillaries is evidence for arteriolar vasoconstriction. Comparing Okamoto and Wistar Kyoto rats, Hutchins (466) found that a greater fraction of the existing arterioles were normally closed in the hypertensive rats, suggesting excessive vasoconstriction in these vessels. The quantitative contribution of vessel rarefaction to total peripheral resistance is not known, but it may not be large. This has been the conclusion of Hallback and colleagues (409).

HORMONES

Measurements of plasma renin activity in Okamoto rats have usually shown normal (43),(505),(840) or low (315),(437) values. Elevated plasma renin activity (221),(853) has occasionally been reported but values were too close to normal to suggest an important role for high renin levels. Bagby and colleagues (43) found normal plasma renin activity in young animals and values of about twice normal in older animals -- when some renal damage might be expected.

There is little evidence of other hormonal abnormalities, although changes in thyroid function have been reported (520).

THE INFLUENCE OF SALT INTAKE

Hypertension develops in the usual manner in animals maintained on a low-sodium diet (24),(602). A high sodium diet, sometimes supplemented with saline, produces additional increases in blood pressure of 20 to 30 mmHg (24),(151),(602),(688),(840) and increased mortality (50).

NEURAL FACTORS

Plasma catecholamine levels have recently been reported as being slightly elevated in this strain (150),(375),(802),(840). Although Lais and colleagues (554) did not see evidence of increased sympathetic nerve activity, there is other experimental support for nervous system involvement in this form of hypertension. Judy and colleagues (491),(492) have observed markedly elevated sympathetic nerve activity in these animals, with blood pressure and nervous activity being proportional. Section of the splanchnic nerves causes a large pressure drop (471) and nerve stimulation of several times normal levels is needed to bring the pressure back to hypertensive levels (471). This data suggests that splanchnic nerve activity is elevated and is making an important contribution to the elevation in blood pressure. However, these data can only be used to demonstrate short-term, in contrast to long-term, influences (472).

Intraventricular 6-hydroxydopamine, shown to prevent hypertension in several other experimental models, also prevents hypertension from developing in the Okamoto rat (260),(288),(399),(545),(721). Intraventricular 6-hydroxydopamine does not decrease pressure in established Okamoto hypertension (399),(545). The response to peripheral sympathectomy is variable, but in general the increase in pressure is slowed somewhat but not stopped (456),(545),(774),(956),(999). Nerve growth factor antiserum has been shown to attenuate the blood pressure increase in Okamoto rats (307),(721). To date then, evidence shows that the nervous system is highly active in these animals but the quantitative contribution of this activity to the long-term pressure increase is still not clear.

RENAL FACTORS

As will be discussed in subsequent chapters, several lines of inquiry have implicated the kidney in the spontaneous hypertension of two other strains of spontaneously hypertensive rats. This could be a congruity of great importance. One experimental approach has been to cross-transplant kidneys in a way that a hypertensive rat receives a normotensive rat's kidney and vice versa. It has been shown in both the Dahl and Bianchi strains that hypertension follows the kidney. With the Okamoto strain, an early and preliminary report indicated that hypertension did not follow the kidney in cross-transplantation (158). Recently, however, a full report has appeared from another laboratory. Kawabe and colleagues (504) back-bred Okamoto and Kyoto control rats one time to improve renal histocompatibility. Kidneys were then transplanted and recipient rats receiving a hypertensive's kidney became hypertensive while recipient rats receiving a normotensive's kidney became normotensive. It is not possible to tell from these studies, however, if the hypertensive's kidney contained an intrinsic, functional defect or if the kidney had been damaged by persistent hypertension of extrarenal origin.

A number of other recent studies have implicated the kidney and the sympathetic nervous system in the genesis of hypertension in Okamoto animals. Liard (586) first reported that renal denervation in young Okamoto rats delayed the onset of hypertension for approximately a month and this observation has subsequently been verified (234), (515),(993). The pressure increase that finally occurs about one month after denervation might be due to reinnervation of the kidneys (993) or to other factors. Reinnervation in normal rats has been shown to begin 1 to 2 weeks after denervation and to be complete in 2 months (516).

The data from transplantation and denervation studies are conflicting in that the former implies an intrinsic renal defect and the latter implies excessive extrinsic influence on the kidneys. If elevated renal nerve traffic was responsible for the hypertension, no transplanted kidneys would be expected to produce hypertension since the sympathetic nerves are severed. If reinnervation did occur, hypertension would be expected to develop in the Okamoto recipient of a Wistar Kyoto kidney and not in the Wistar Kyoyto recipient of an Okamoto kidney. The latter has been observed and this question remains unresolved.

Several other studies have established neural and/or renal abnormalities. Renal sympathetic nerve activity is increased (491). An increased renal vascular responsiveness to sympathetic nerve activity (174) and infused norepinephrine (175) have been reported. Fink and Brody (290), however, found elevated renal resistance but no evidence of unusual sympathetic influence on the kidneys.

Detailed renal function studies have shown renal vasoconstriction (28),(40), normal or low renal blood flow (28),(40), and normal autoregulatory responses. Folkow and colleagues (364),(308) have reported that renal resistance is elevated in this model when the kidneys are maximally dilated. Renal resistance is also elevated with normal perfusion (290) and the primary site of vasoconstriction appears to be the afferent arteriole

(40),(364). The analogy to the effectiveness of the Goldblatt clamp in the same region in producing hypertension cannot be overlooked, but autoregulatory renal vasoconstriction is also the normal physiological response to an elevated renal perfusion pressure. Therefore, it is not clear if elevated renal resistance is causing hypertension or if hypertension is causing elevated renal resistance.

DiBona and Rios (226) found that arterial pressure had to be elevated in order to obtain normal sodium excretion from the Okamoto kidney. This suggests that increased renal perfusion pressure is needed to maintain regular salt and water balance by offsetting the increased autonomic influence or other antinatriuretic tendencies present in these kidneys.

CHAPTER 15

GENETIC HYPERTENSION: THE DAHL SUBSTRAINS OF SALT-SENSITIVE AND SALT-RESISTANT RATS

The two Dahl or Brookhaven substrains of rats were developed by inbreeding at the Brookhaven National Laboratories in the 1960's. They have been named "salt-sensitive" and "salt-resistant" since one becomes hypertensive when placed on a sodium-rich diet while the other remains normotensive.

The most striking differences between these two substrains have been found in the kidneys. The evidence points to a causal role for renal dysfunction in the hypertension of the "salt-sensitive" substrain. This substrain shows some narrowing of the renal arteries and decreased medullary blood flow even before the hypertension-producing, salt-rich diet has been started. After hypertension has developed, further renal vasoconstriction has been observed and the excretory capability of the kidney is suppressed. When kidneys from hypertensive "salt-sensitive" rats are transplanted to normotensive "salt-resistant" recipients, hypertension develops. Conversely, when kidneys from normotensive "salt-resistant" rats are transplanted to hypertensive "salt-sensitive" rats, normotension results.

Non-renal factors have also been studied. Several aspects of vascular responsiveness in the "salt-sensitive" substrain are increased. Observed biochemical abnormalities involve adrenal enzymes and unusual proteins found in colloidal material in the pituitary cleft of the "salt-resistant" substrain. This last factor is probably not related to blood pressure control.

THE ORIGIN OF DAHL OR BROOKHAVEN SALT-SENSITIVE RATS

Lewis Dahl was intensely interested throughout his career in the role of salt in the genesis of hypertension and he invested considerable effort in developing and maintaining two complimentary substrains of rats (203). One of these substrains remains normotensive with normal sodium intake but becomes markedly hypertensive when given salt-rich diet. Because of this it has been called a "salt-sensitive" substrain. The other substrain remains normotensive on normal and salt-rich diets and it has therefore been called a "salt-resistant" substrain. Diets with a very high sodium content have been used. Hypertension persists even after the salt-rich diet is discontinued (206).

HEMODYNAMICS

Ganguli and colleagues (337) observed an increase in cardiac output in the "salt-sensitive" strain when a salt-rich diet was instituted. Flow returned to normal as hypertension became fully developed. These transients could be interpreted as an autoregulatory response, except that "salt-resistant" animals showed the same response without developing hypertension. A possible explanation is that the two substrains have quite different autoregulatory responses to overperfusion.

Exchangeable sodium is normal in "salt-sensitive" rats with established hypertension (829).

HORMONES

A humoral explanation for the development of hypertension in Dahl rats has long been sought, but with little success. Plasma renin activity appears to be less than normal in "salt-sensitive" animals (478),(783). Rapp and colleagues (783) have investigated additional endocrine factors. Plasma aldosterone is low in the "salt-sensitive" animal. Corticosterone and deoxycorticostrone are normal. 18-hydroxy-deoxycorticosterone is elevated and is genetically linked to increased 18-hydroxylase activity (779). While 18-hydroxy-deoxycorticosterone could be making a large contribution to the observed hypertension, the results of cross-breeding experiments indicate that only 16% of the total blood pressure increase is directly attributable to this steroid (781).

Rapp and colleagues (778),(780) have discovered some unusual proteins in the pituitary of "salt-resistant" Dahl rats. These proteins have been genetically linked to blood pressure. However, the physiological role of these proteins remains unknown and it is likely that they are not directly involved in the etiology of the hypertension

(782). It is more likely that the genetic control of synthesis of these proteins and the genetic control of arterial pressure come from the same region or adjacent sites on an important chromosome.

NEURAL FACTORS

There is some evidence for an increased influence of the sympathetic nervous system on blood pressure in "salt-sensitive" rats. Enhanced constriction of the hindquarters with sympathetic nerve stimulation (909), increased renal sensitivity to norepinephrine (293) and exaggerated vasodilation with splanchnic nerve section (909) have been reported. Neonatal sympathectomy by guanethidine prevents hypertension in "salt-sensitive" rats (324) as does peripheral sympathectomy with 6-hydroxydopamine (912).

Imposed stresses result in higher blood pressure in "salt-sensitive" rats than in "salt-resistant" rats (321),(323).

RENAL FACTORS

A renal abnormality has been observed by Jaffe *et al* (480) in the "salt-sensitive" substrain even before excess salt is administered and hypertension develops. An invagination into the lumen is seen in the afferent vasculature at the junction between the arcuate artery and afferent arteriole. After salt administration and the development of hypertension, this invagination becomes extremely severe and it appears that a tortuous vasoconstriction has developed in the blood supply to the glomerulus.

Further evidence for renal involvement comes from kidney cross-transplantation studies (202),(205). Transplanting the kidney from a normotensive "salt-resistant" animal into a "salt-sensitive" hypertensive animal results in normotension in the "salt-sensitive" animal. Conversely, transplantation of the kidney from a "salt-sensitive" hypertensive animal to a "salt-resistant" recipient produces hypertension in the "salt-resistant" and previously normotensive recipient. These results are summarized below.

SYSTOLIC BLOOD PRESSURE (mmHg)
FOLLOWING KIDNEY TRANSPLANTATION (202)

	Salt-Resistant Substrain	Salt-Sensitive Substrain
No Transplant	132	186
Received Resistant Kidney	132	123
No Transplant	128	167
Received Sensitive Kidney	155	167

Interpretation of pressure changes after transplantation are complicated by the possibility that kidneys from hypertensive animals may have sustained pressure-induced damage before transplantation.

Tobian and colleagues (935) have removed the kidneys from the two Dahl substrains and studied their capacity for salt and water excretion when isolated and perfused. The kidneys from the hypertensive "salt-sensitive" strain excrete much less salt and water at any perfusion pressure than the "salt-resistant" normotensive strain. When the kidneys from the hypertensive animal are perfused at normotensive pressures, only minimal amounts of salt and water are excreted. Hence, it would appear that an increase in perfusion pressure is needed to maintain salt and water balance in these animals, although many of the particulars are still not known. Tobian et al (936) have more recently reported that the cause of impaired natriuresis is not located in the kidneys of "salt-sensitive" rats but in their blood. Hence, when a kidney from a "salt-resistant" rat is perfused by "salt-sensitive" blood, impaired sodium excretion is observed. This result is in direct conflict with the renal transplantation data cited above and the matter currently remains unresolved.

Fink et al (293) observed that the "salt sensitive" substrain had a lower renal vascular resistance than the "salt-resistant" substrain before a high-salt diet was instituted. But with excess dietary salt, the "salt-resistant" kidney responded by vasodilating while the "salt-sensitive" kidney did not. It appears that the "salt-sensitive" kidney does not have the excretory capacity to handle large sodium loads while the "salt-resistant" kidney does.

Ganguli and colleagues (336) have observed decreased blood flow in the renal papilla in "salt-sensitive" rats both before and after hypertension developed. The significance of this observation is not known.

One additional observation will be mentioned. In a previous chapter, the role of the contralateral kidney in two-kidney Goldblatt hypertension was discussed. It was suggested that the excretory function of this kidney is a very important part of the genesis of hypertension in the two-kidney model. The "salt-sensitive" substrain has kidneys which are potentially salt-retaining while the "salt-resistant" substrain has kidneys which are potentially very good salt excreters. Dahl *et al* (204) demonstrated that when these two substrains were used in two-kidney Goldblatt preparation, the "salt-sensitive" substrain developed a much higher arterial pressure than did the "salt-resistant" substrain. One interpretation of this is as follows: after clamping, the "salt-sensitive" strain requires a high arterial pressure to achieve salt and water balance by way of an unclamped, contralateral kidney which does not have particularly good excretory function. In contrast, the "salt-resistant" strain uses the contralateral kidney to maintain salt and water balance at a much lower pressure after clamping because this kidney has particularly good excretory function.

CHAPTER 16

GENETIC HYPERTENSION: OTHER MODELS

Rats, mice, and even turkeys have been selectively inbred to alter blood pressure. The primary use of many of these models has been to study the inheritance of specific traits rather than the physiology of blood pressure control. However, blood pressure control has been studied in two inbred strains of hypertensive rats in addition to the Okamoto and Dahl strains.

The New Zealand strain was developed in the late 1950's and was thus the first strain of genetically hypertensive rats. But, it has not been studied widely outside of New Zealand and the cause of the hypertension remains unknown. Plasma renin activity and sodium metabolism appear to be normal. Some indications of sympathetic overactivity have been found.

The Bianchi or Milan strain of genetically hypertensive rats was developed by inbreeding in Italy it the late 1960's. It has primarily been studied by the originators of the strain, who first demonstrated the possibility of renal cross-transplantation in the rat. It was then demonstrated that the chronic level of blood pressure after renal cross-transplantation was determined by the kidney, not the recipient.

THE DEVELOPMENT OF GENETIC HYPERTENSION IN SEVERAL DIFFERENT SPECIES

Selective inbreeding has been employed in attempts to alter blood pressure in mice (837), rats, rabbits (11), chickens (897), turkeys (543), and other species. These studies have shown: firstly that pressure can be altered by inbreeding, secondly that pressure is under polygenic control, and thirdly that Mendelian dominance is not observed in blood pressure changes of genetic origin. A comprehensive review has been provided by Schlager (836).

The physiological basis of blood pressure increases and decreases has not been explored in most of these species.

But, in addition to the Okamoto and Dahl strains of rats, two other strains have been studied from a physiological viewpoint and are discussed further below.

THE NEW ZEALAND STRAIN OF GENETIC HYPERTENSIVE RATS

New Zealand hypertensive rats are often described as having "genetic" hypertension to help distinguish them from Okamoto rats with "spontaneous" hypertension. The New Zealand strain was originally developed in the laboratory of Professor Smirk and in 1958 it was the first strain of spontaneously hypertensive rats to be described (879). At first the incidence of hypertension was reported to be less than 100 percent but continued inbreeding has apparently improved this incidence to the full 100 percent level. The strain has remained primarily in New Zealand and has been studied extensively by investigators in Dunedin. Recently, Simpson and colleagues (866) have summarized these investigations.

Hemodynamics

Cardiac output has been reported to be normal in this model (134). Renal blood flow may be reduced a little bit (130).

Plasma volume, extracellular fluid volume, and total body water are normal (370) in young New Zealand rats that are in the process of becoming hypertensive. Plasma and extracellular fluid volume are low (369),(569),(568) in adult animals. Hematocrit is increased (369),(569). These data offer no support for the idea that volume expansion is playing a role in the genesis of the hypertension. But, the observation that venous compliance is decreased (863) complicates interpretation of the volume data.

Hormones

Plasma renin activity is a little low in this model (368),(569). No other hormones have been implicated.

Neural factors

Evidence for a nervous component in this genetic model

comes from several different experimental protocols. Firstly, peripheral sympathectomy by 6-hydroxydopamine (154),(156) or antiserum to nerve growth factor (153) prevents full development of hypertension. However, blood pressure remained higher in treated hypertensives than in comparably treated controls in these experiments. Hexamethonium decreased blood pressure to a lower level in New Zealand hypertensive rats than in renal hypertensive rats (757); even lower levels of pressure were seen, however, in control animals given hexamethonium. Stimulation of the sympathetic nerves caused a greater pressor response in hypertensive animals than in normotensive controls (660). In total, these data support, somewhat indirectly, a neurogenic component in New Zealand hypertension.

Renal factors

There is some evidence for a renal defect in this model. Recent studies have indicated that while glomerular filtration is close to normal there is reduced renal blood flow (130) and redistribution of flow within the kidney. Redistribution is away from the cortex (130) and in some other instances such redistribution has been associated with decreased sodium excretion (451),(638),(766).

THE BIANCHI OR MILAN STRAIN OF SPONTANEOUSLY HYPERTENSIVE RATS

The Bianchi or Milan strain was derived from Wistar rats in 1964 by Professor Bianchi in Milan, Italy (85). This model has not been widely circulated, but it has been extensively investigated in Professor Bianchi's laboratories (80),(78). The strain develops a mild hypertension and shows a number of hemodynamic and renal abnormalities when compared to a companion normotensive control strain. These data have recently been summarized (78).

Hemodynamics

No differences in cardiac output were observed when Milan hypertensive and normotensive rats were compared (410). Measurements of exchangable sodium and of salt and water balance show sodium retention in young hypertensive animals as the high blood pressure is developing (79), (83).

Hormones

Compared to normotensive controls, plasma renin activity has been shown to be decreased in young animals and normal in adults (79),(83). No other hormones have been implicated in the genesis of hypertension.

Neural factors

Hallback *et al* (410) found that heart rate was decreased in Milan rats and the response to imposed stress was normal. They concluded that the Milan strain showed less evidence of neural involvement in hypertension than the Okamoto strain of hypertensive rats.

Renal factors

An examination of the development of the kidney in this strain shows that the adult hypertensive rat has fewer nephrons than its normotensive counterpart (41). Younger rats show decreased whole-kidney glomerular filtration rate and single nephron glomerular filtration rate (41).

Strong evidence for the involvement of the kidney in this strain of hypertensive rats comes from cross transplantation studies (83),(84). As in the Dahl strain, it has been shown that the transplantation of a normotensive kidney to a hypertensive animal results in normalization of blood pressure, while transplantation of a hypertensive kidney to a normotensive rat results in hypertension. Transplants between young animals that did not have fully developed hypertension showed somewhat similar results (84). It appears that the kidney helps to sustain hypertension in the Milan strain and that it also has a causal role in the pressure increase before any pressure-induced renal damage might develop.

Bianchi *et al* (78) have suggested that a decrease in capillary permeability, in the kidney and in the systemic circulation, might elevate arterial pressure and account for the observed hemodynamic and renal peculiarities.

CHAPTER 17

THE PHYSIOLOGY OF ESSENTIAL HYPERTENSION

Most human hypertension does not show obvious physiological abnormalities and such cases are called "essential" or "idiopathic." Rigorous experimental investigation is not often possible, and consequently an acceptable explanation for the cause of essential hypertension has not been developed.

Some physiological abnormalities have been found, but often the measured values are quite close to normal. Plasma renin activity is usually normal or low, and renin release is often sluggish. Cardiac output is elevated in some young hypertensives; flow decreases with age. Fluid volumes are normal to low. Venous compliance is decreased. Plasma catecholamines are close to normal, but the response to acute stress may be greater than normal. Baroreceptor responsiveness is attenuated. The kidney shows progressive decreases in flow and filtration and increases in filtration fraction.

Many different single causes of essential hypertension have been postulated and it has also been suggested that essential hypertension is actually a composite disease with many causes. But, less diversity is also a possibility. If inferences are drawn from animals having experimental or genetic hypertension of known origin, its possible that essential hypertension is caused by a genetic deficiency in renal function that is amplified by excessive sodium intake and/or overactivity of the sympathetic nervous system. Recalling the efficacy of the Goldblatt clamp in elevating blood pressure, an usually high afferent renal resistance might be the real culprit.

EPIDEMIOLOGICAL vs PHYSIOLOGICAL CONSIDERATIONS

Hypertension is said to exist when systolic and/or diastolic pressures pass above arbitrarily defined upper limits of normalcy, as discussed in a previous chapter. When there is no obvious reason for the pressure increase, essential or idiopathic hypertension is said to exist.

The epidemiology of human hypertension has also been discussed in a previous chapter. Studies comparing different societies and studies within societies have at times shown that the prevalence of hypertension can be correlated with age, obesity, sodium intake, and genetic and familial factors. None of these correlations indicate what mechanism or mechanisms might be causing the increased vascular resistance.

Essential hypertension has been most difficult to study experimentally. Arterial pressure may increase in an individual slowly and insidiously over several decades; prospective studies designed to follow such increases risk being tedious, expensive, and beyond the interests of most scientists and agencies supplying funds for medical research. Highly invasive studies are not acceptable for humane reasons. Data must be normalized to accomodate a wide range of body sizes and shapes. The proven benefits of antihypertensive therapy makes it very difficult to justify extended periods of observation using unmedicated hypertensives.

Theoretically, the most attractive experimental approach is the longitudinal study. Repeated measurements are made on a single individual and time-dependent features in the progression of hypertension are captured. Two less demanding alternatives are cross-sectional and retrospective studies. In the cross-sectional approach, measurements are made on many different subjects with the assumption that isolated measurements using many subjects will eventually show the same trends as multiple measurements using a few subjects. In the retrospective approach, subjects with fully established hypertension are identified and past medical records are reviewed to see if any striking features emerge. All of these experimental strategies have contributed to our meager understanding of the physiological aspects of essential hypertension.

PHYSIOLOGICAL STUDIES

The renin-angiotensin system

The mean values of plasma renin activity (33),(121), (372) and plasma angiotensin II concentration (58), (334) are normal in essential hypertension, but the distribution is broad enough so that single individuals may show high, normal or low levels. Schalekamp and colleagues

(832),(833) have studied trends in plasma renin activity with increasing age and severity of hypertension. A biphasic response was observed in which plasma renin activity decreased with progressive increases in renal vascular resistance; with very severe hypertension, plasma renin activity increased to become much greater than normal. It appears that plasma renin activity is relatively normal in benign hypertension and decreases with age just as in normotensives. But when renal resistance is very high, renin secretion rates increase just as they do in many other forms of renal disease.

Plasma renin activity is very sensitive to changes in sodium intake, with large increases occurring during sodium restriction and suppression to unmeasurable levels occurring during excessive salt intake. Brunner, Laragh, and colleagues (121),(125),(560) have emphasized this fact and have noted that sodium intake must be known before subtle abnormalities in renin levels can be identified in hypertensive subjects. Antihypertensive drugs, such as beta-adrenergic antagonists and diuretics, can also have a marked influence on plasma renin activity. Comparison among individual hypertensives or groups of hypertensive must be undertaken with caution.

The responsiveness of the renin-angiotensin system in essential hypertension is often less than that seen in normotensive subjects (68),(197),(446),(521),(535),(942). Renin increases with upright posture and in response to diuretic administration have been shown to be attenuated, particularly in those hypertensive subjects with low resting renin levels. Suppression of renin by volume expansion has also been snown to be less than normal (942). Neither the reason for this nor the importance in the pathogenesis of essential hypertension are clear. However, attenuated responsiveness suggests that the mechanisms that control renin release are misjudging changes in the salt and water stores of the body.

Hemodynamics

Possibly 10% of young adults will show mild and/or occasional blood pressure elevations. Accordingly, this has been labeled borderline or labile hypertension. There are indications of sympathetic overactivity and one-third or more of these subjects present a "hyperdynamic" circulation (494),(819). Cardiac output and heart rate are elevated (254),(493),(818), (819),(985). Oxygen consumption is also elevated (493), and increases in metabolic rate may be the underlying cause of the increased cardiac output. Peripheral resistance is not necessarily elevated. Blood and plasma volumes are normal (818) or decreased (257),(496),(819) while central blood volume is increased (257). Plasma renin activity is variable but on the average, normal (262),(263),(265). Elevated levels have been associated with sympathetic overactivity (262),(265). Autonomic activity is often increased but the manifestations are highly variable (494). Increased sympathetic nerve activity (263), increased beta-adrenergic activity (495), increased beta-adrenergic receptor sensitivity (328) and decreased parasympathetic activity (495) have all been implicated at different times.

Borderline or labile hypertension probably represents only a temporary increase in arterial pressure linked to abnormal neural and possibly psychological (264) factors. The majority of subjects with borderline hypertension do not go on to develop sustained essential hypertension (578). Therefore, it is likely that the temporary pressure increases of borderline hypertension and the gradual, persistent pressure increases of essential hypertension involved somewhat different mechanisms.

In contrast to borderline hypertension, blood flow is not elevated in well-established essential hypertension. Pickering (758) reached this conclusion in 1935 after measuring blood flow in the arm. Since then, many studies have shown that cardiac output is normal (47),(90),(110),(330), (814),(816),(818). Flow decreases with age just as it does in normotensives (90). The data of Safar and Milliez is summarized on the next page.

Peripheral resistance is definitely elevated in established essential hypertension. This elevation, relative to normotensive subjects, is maintained even at maximum vasodilation (182),(305),(874),(875). Increased minimum resistance is thought to be due to structural changes in the peripheral vasculature (303),(304). This abnormality slowly disappears with successful antihypertensive therapy (873). Takeshita and Mark (911) have recently reported that minimum vascular resistance is also increased in 25 year old subjects with borderline hypertension. There are several possible interpretations. One is that vascular restructuring can occur very rapidly. Another is that vascular restructuring is not a direct consequence of persistent elevations in pressure and that it might, in fact, precede pressure elevations.

Measurement of blood, plasma, and extracellular fluid volumes shows these variables to be normal or low in essential hypertension (52),(115),(330),(443),(534),(814),(816),(818),(918),(930) with one exception (381). The smallest volumes occur at the highest arterial pressures (146),(251),(943). These observations and others provide strong evidence against a primary expansion of fluid volume during the development of essential hypertension. But in some cases uncertainty has been added by the normalization procedures used, since volumes do not vary in direct proportion to body weight (273).

HEMODYNAMICS IN BORDERLINE
AND PERMANENT HYPERTENSION (818)

	Normotension	Hypertension Borderline	Hypertension Permanent
Mean Arterial Pressure (mmHg)	86	105	145
Cardiac Index (l/min/m.m)	3.15	4.09	3.29
Total Peripheral Resistance	2221	2099	3661
Heart Rate (beats/min)	72	80	79
Blood Volume (ml/kg)	76	77	75

Analysis of pulsatile arterial pressure and flow indicates that arterial compliance is reduced in essential hypertension (861). Plethysmographic measurements in arms and digits show evidence of decreased venous compliance in borderline (910) and established (2),(133),(864),(971) essential hypertension. A less direct but possibly more functional estimate of venous compliance comes from observing the response of central venous pressure to volume expansion. In 1962, Hejl and colleagues (429) first showed that saline infusion produced an abnormally large increase in cardiac output in essential hypertensives. Ulrych et al (945) then showed that this response was coupled to abnormal increases in venous pressure; this data indicated that venous compliance was decreased. Ulrych's observation has recently been confirmed by Safar and colleagues (599),(815). Using dextran infusion, they found decreased venous compliance with normal cardiac function. Pressures on the venous side of the circulation seem to be slightly elevated in essential hypertension (274),(599),(815).

The hemodynamic influence of blood volume changes depends heavily on the vascular compliance in which the volume reside. Until procedures are developed to quantitatively evaluate the combined volume-compliance changes, it will not be known if subjects with decreased volume and compliance are functionally underhydrated, functionally normally hydrated, or functionally overhydrated. The Okomoto strain of spontaneously hypertensive rats show similar tendencies and measurement of mean circulatory filling pressure in these animals has revealed a definite functional overhydration (824). Safar and colleagues (816) reached precisely the same conclusion for human essential hypertension using extrapolation techniques of questionable value.

Neural factors

There has been considerable interest in the possible importance of the sympathetic nervous system in essential hypertension. In 1973, Louis and colleagues (601) reported a direct correlation between plasma catecholamines and arterial pressure in patients with essential hypertension. Since that time many other laboratories have measured plasma norepinephrine and epinephrine but the results are equivocal. In some instances normal catecholamine levels have been reported in essential hypertension (468),(488),(555),(750),(919),(964),(979). In other instances increased catecholamine levels have been observed (215),(223),(259),(457),(601),(854). These results are tempered by the observations that 1) hypertensive subjects are often older than normotensive control subjects and 2) plasma catecholamines increase with age in both normotensives and hypertensives (555),(979). After adjustment for age, the evidence that catecholamines are increased in essential hypertension is much weaker. Plasma catecholamine levels in essential hypertension are, of course, always far less than those seen in pheochromocytoma.

Jones and colleagues (488) have examined the procedures used in selecting control subjects for catecholamine determinations. They found that normotensive and hypertensive outpatients showed identical plasma norepinephrine levels while laboratory personnel used to generate "normal" control data showed lower concentrations; presumably the latter were more comfortable with the protocols and setting.

Small increases in circulating catecholamines are not easily interpreted. The direct vasoconstrictor effect of low levels of circulating catecholamines *per se* is likely to be small. But, if increased plasma levels result directly from transmitter spillover from adrenergic nerve endings, then moderately elevated blood levels could be symptomatic of large and important increases in sympathetic nerve activity.

A very approximate quantitative analysis of the interrelationships between sympathetic nerve activity, circulating norepinephrine and blood pressure is possible. The data of Planz and Planz (763) indicates that 90% or more of circulating norepinephrine is spilled neurotransmitter rather than an adrenal secretion. From the data of Mathias *et al* (628), it appears that, very roughly, an increase in sympathetic activity that acutely raises arterial pressure by 20 mmHg will spill enough norepinephrine into the circulation to double plasma norepinephrine levels. Blood levels of neurotransmitter represent a vasoconstriction that is about 20-30 times as great as that produced directly by circulating norepinephrine. Therefore, the small increases in plasma catecholamines sometimes seen in essential hypertension warrant careful consideration.

Predominately qualitative studies of basal sympathetic nerve activity in essential hypertensives have shown some evidence of baroreceptor resetting but no other peculiarities (969),(970). Sympatholytic drugs have not been as effective in lowering blood pressure in essential hypertension as would be expected in straightforward cases of sympathetically mediated vasoconstriction.

In contrast to normal basal catecholamine levels, a pattern of abnormal sympathetic function emerges when patients with essential hypertension are stressed. Provocative stimuli, including difficult mental tasks and threatening encounters, produce greater blood pressure increases in essential hypertensives than normotensives (108),(109),(428), (691),(828),(855). Pressure increases are accompanied by evidence of excessive vasoconstriction and sympathetic overactivity.

Abnormally large responses to extrinsic stimuli might be related to inadequate baroreceptor function. Non-invasive measurement of total baroreceptor function is not possible, but a method devised by Smyth and colleagues (883) characterizes the component involved in heart rate control. Angiotensin or phenylephrine injections temporarily elevate arterial pressure without directly affecting heart rate. The resultant bradycardia is used as a quantitative measure of baroreceptor responsiveness. This method has uniformly shown depressed baroreflex responsiveness in established essential hypertension (371),(531),(614),(777), (862),(913),(977). Eckberg (253) used neck suction to stimulate the baroreceptors and found normal reflex responsiveness in mild borderline hypertensives but depressed values in more severe borderline hypertension. Takeshita _et al_ (913) found that borderline hypertensives had a _depressed_ responsiveness that was midway between the values seen in normotensives and established hypertensives. The implication is that decreased responsiveness accompanies rather than follows the development of hypertension. This latter data does not support the notion that decreased baroreceptor responsiveness in established hypertension is secondary to slowly developing pressure-induced modifications of the walls of the large arteries.

Sleight (877) has suggested that inadequate reflex control of arterial pressure might actually be the cause of essential hypertension, but verification of this concept will undoubtedly be difficult. When baroreceptor function is interrupted by surgical methods in experimental animals, the lability of arterial pressure increases to a much greater extent than what is seen in essential hypertension. Instead of decreased reflex responsiveness, hypertension would be more likely to result from an upward displacement of the normal functional range of the baroreceptors to higher pressure levels. But, the baroreceptors have been shown to adapt in experimental hypertension and they may also adapt in essential hypertension (253),(531); theoretically, causal _and_ compensatory changes in baroreceptor function would _be_ expected to be nearly identical and first causes would hardly be distinguishable from secondary effects.

In addition to alterations in neurophysiological function, specific psychological features have been linked with essential hypertension. The patient with essential hypertension has been characterized as being outwardly calm, friendly and eager to please while inwardly he represses strong emotions, hostility and aggressiveness (213),(667),(981),(995). He may be wary, tense, scared or lack confidence. The studies that led to this characterization have included a certain degree of subjectivity, of course. It is not clear whether this particular psychological stereotype should be thought of as a cause of or a consequence of elevated pressure.

Renal factors

Renal blood flow and glomerular filtration rate decrease with age (212),(448). They also decrease with increasing severity of hypertension (69),(249),(212),(320),(354),(448),(751),(792),(816). Flow decreases somewhat faster than filtration and the calculated filtration fraction, therefore, increases. Hollenberg and associates (446),(449) found that renal blood flow was slightly greater than normal in some subjects with mild hypertension but less than normal in the majority with mild hypertension and in those with more severe hypertension.

Decreased flow at increased perfusing pressure signals renal vasoconstriction. This constriction seems to be more functional than fixed before advanced nephrosclerosis sets in. Exaggerated renal dilation has been observed in essential hypertensives during infusion of vasodilating drugs (447) and saline (603). The afferent artery appears to be the site of vasoconstriction (170),(356),(603) and, as in Goldblatt hypertension, this could have an important effect on blood pressure .

The question of whether decreases in renal blood flow are the cause of hypertension or a consequence of it remains unanswered. For instance, Hollenberg and colleagues (450) found that most cases of decreased renal blood flow were accompanied by evidence of vascular damage. In contrast, Safar and colleagues (814) have found a strong negative correlation between arterial pressure and renal blood flow without evidence of renal damage. A detailed description of the renal circulation in hypertension has been provided by Hollenberg and Adams (446).

The excretion of water, electrolytes and filtered metabolites remains roughly normal in essential hypertension. This excretion occurs, however, at a renal perfusion pressure which is greater than normal. It had remained a point of speculation for some time as to whether or not the kidneys in essential hypertension would function properly when perfused at normotensive levels.

Recently, Omvik *et al* (715) lowered arterial pressure in hypertensives using nitroprusside and showed that excretion was markedly depressed in these subjects as renal perfusion pressure approached normotensive levels. The cause of this decrease in excretory function is not known, but such deficiencies could play an important role in the genesis of essential hypertension. Decreases in renal excretory capacity could also be secondary to persistent elevations in arterial pressure (450).

LOW-RENIN ESSENTIAL HYPERTENSION

Traditionally, overactivity of the renin-angiotensin system was judged to be a likely cause of essential hypertension. The fact gradually emerged that some patients with essential hypertension show resting plasma renin activities that are below normal and depressed responsiveness when renin release is stimulated. It was then suspected that a separate and special type of hypertension had been identified and this was called "low-renin" essential hypertension. An excellent review is provided by Dunn and Tannen (248).

Hypertension with low plasma renin activity suggests mineralocorticoid excess, as in primary aldosteronism. Normal or slightly expanded fluid volumes and normal plasma aldosterone levels have been reported (248). Since most values are very close to normal, in comparison to primary aldosteronism again, any pertubations seem to be far smaller than what might be required to produce hypertension. Similarly, plasma potassium levels can be severely depressed in primary aldosteronism while they are essentially normal in low-renin hypertension. Patients with low-renin hypertension respond very favorably to diuretics and spironolactone (248).

It may be that an unfamiliar humoral-volume pattern developes in low-renin hypertension because of over-secretion of some relatively unknown steroid. Several candidates, intermediary compounds in steroid synthesis (592),(640) have been considered but current evidence is not conclusive. Baxter and colleagues (54) used an assay built around mineralocorticoid receptors and could find no evidence of unusual mineralocorticoid activity in plasma from low-renin subjects.

The levels of blood pressure seen in low-renin hypertension are the same as or greater than those in normal or high-renin hypertension. This indicates that low-renin hypertension is not just a mild form of essential hypertension. It has been claimed that those with low-renin hypertension show decreased morbidity and mortality (121), but there is a considerable amount of data that demonstrates no correlation between renin levels and morbid events (15),(245),(831).

Plasma renin activities range from low to high in essential hypertension without discontinuity (33),(121),(372). Taking all available data into consideration, it doesn't seem likely that low-renin hypertension is a special variant of essential hypertension caused by excessive secretion of some steroid. It's more likely that plasma renin activity and responsiveness tend to be a little low in all of essential hypertension unless there is concomitant volume contraction, renal damage or increased sympathetic activity. This would account for the observed spectrum of plasma renin activities.

THE CAUSE OF ESSENTIAL HYPERTENSION

As the studies cited above indicate, a diversity of usually small peculiarities have been observed in hypertensive subjects. These observations coupled with comparable diversity seen in epidemiological studies suggest that hypertension is not one disease but a variety of diseases. In 1949, Page (730) presented a mosiac theory of hypertension which was more of a philosophical overview than a rigorous theory. The idea: Many different factors influence arterial pressure and therefore many different factors can be responsible for the development of essential hypertension.

The mosaic theory may be an accurate statement of the case. However, there are several worrisome aspects to this contention. One is that if a great many factors can influence arterial pressure, then the long-term control of blood pressure is likely to be very poor. We know however that arterial pressure is remarkably stable in man and animals over the long run. For instance, increases in plasma catecholamines and plasma renin activity are considered potential causes of essential hypertension. Yet, fluctuations in these two variables are commonly much greater than the fluctuations observed in arterial pressure. A second consideration is that if there are a wide variety of causes of essential hypertension, few correlations would emerge when unselected groups of hypertensive subjects are studied. But, some definite although admittedly subtle correlations have been emerging and this suggests that essential hypertension is not the result of a broad spectrum of causes. Of course, the correlations that do emerge could be entirely due to factors that are secondary to the blood pressure increase.

A slightly different view is that essential hypertension results from one primary cause. Environmental influences such as excessive sodium intake or unusual psychological stresses would not normally cause hypertension but would exacerbate the underlying slow-but-sure hypertensive process. In this scheme, hypertension would develop in those with the requisite genetic background even in favorable environmental circumstances. But, adverse environmental influences would increase the prevalence of hypertension. Clinical and physiological evidence would be varied but not totally random.

There is not enough evidence available to reach firm conclusions as to the cause of essential hypertension. However, speculation can use data from experimental animal models. Firstly, many forms of experimental hypertension involve some manipulation of the kidneys or excessive external influences on renal function. Therefore, the kidneys might be the place to look for a cause of essential hypertension. Secondly, the Okomoto strain of spontaneously hypertensive rats bears some striking similarities to human essential hypertension. The blood pressure increase in these animals depends on their pedigree. This strain shows as few physiological abnormalities as patients with essential hypertension; in fact, since the creation of the Okamoto strain the physiological basis of its hypertension has been as hotly debated as have the causes of essential hypertension. There is evidence, however, that the Okamoto strain and other strains of spontaneously hypertensive rats have a renal abnormality that is directly related to the development of hypertension. Thirdly, the Dahl strains of spontaneously hypertensive rats illustrate the importance of a genetic predisposition to the development of hypertension. The salt-sensitive substrain develops hypertension when salt intake is high. The salt-resistant substrain does not get hypertensive even when the salt intake is high. These observations in total suggest that there might be a genetically-related renal defect in essential hypertension (170) but the needed supporting evidence is missing.

CHAPTER 18

ANTIHYPERTENSIVE THERAPY

It has traditionally been thought, but only recently demonstrated conclusively, that interventions which lower blood pressure also lower morbidity and mortality. Confirmation comes from successful and regular use of a variety of antihypertensive drugs that were first introduced in the 1950's and 60's. The antihypertensive agents that are currently in use or under consideration can be roughly grouped according to mechanisms of action as : diuretics and natriuretics, beta-adrenergic receptor blockers, sympatholytics and drugs that act on the central nervous system, direct vasodilators, and converting enzyme inhibitors or angiotensin antagonists. The last group will be discussed in detail in the following chapter.

A BRIEF HISTORY OF ANTIHYPERTENSIVE THERAPY

It has been suggested that U. S. President Franklin Delano Roosevelt died in 1945 of malignant hypertension just a short time before suitable antihypertensive drugs came into use (176). At the time, salt restriction and sedatives were about all that was available. In contrast, in the 1950's and 60's a wealth of new drugs came into widespread clinical use.

Alkaloids extracted from *Rauwolfia serpentina* had been shown to reduce blood pressure in India in the 1930's and 40's but use was sporadic. Reserpine was isolated from *Rauwolfia* in 1952 (681) and was later synthesized. A potent antihypertensive agent had finally become available.

In 1950 Reubi (791) reported that hydralazine was a vasodilator and that it lowered blood pressure in man. In 1957, Freis and Wilson (319) and Hollander and Wilkins (445) demonstrated the clinical effectiveness of chlorothiazide. In the same year, the diuretic properties of spironolactone were also demonstrated (498). In 1959 the initial clinical use of guanethidine was reported by Page and Dustan (732). Oates and colleagues showed that alpha-methyldopa would lower blood pressure in 1960 (706). In 1962, diazoxide was shown to have antihypertensive properties even though the diuretic response produced by similarly structured compounds was missing in this case (809). In 1964 Prichard and Gillam (770) reported that propranolol was antihypertensive.

In the past decade, many additional antihypertensive agents have been approved for routine use or are currently undergoing evaluation.

THE HAZARDS OF HYPERTENSION

It has been known since antiquity that high blood pressure increases morbidity and mortality. Confirmation in quantitative terms has come from the records of life insurance companies. The following table shows survival rates over 5 to 20 years for 45 year old men with no known disease (580).

LONGEVITY AS A FUNCTION OF BLOOD PRESSURE
(45 Year Old Males)

Blood Pressure (mmHg)	Percent Surviving After 5 Yrs	10 Yrs	15 Yrs	20 Yrs
132/85	96	91	84	75
142/90	95	87	78	66
152/95	93	83	71	56
162/100	90	78	63	46

A firm connection between high blood pressure and increasing morbidity and mortality has also been seen in studies that have sampled suitably large segments of a population for statistical analysis. For instance, the Framingham study, begun in 1949 in the Massachusett's town of that name, has followed over 5000 subjects. These studies show a strong correlation between high blood pressure and the incidence of coronary artery and heart disease (501),(940), nephrosclerosis and renal failure (363), and infarction and aneurism in the brain and in the large arteries in general (361). Hypertension accelerates the development of atherosclerosis, as demonstrated in experimental animals (666) and clinical studies (361).

The exact connection between elevated blood pressure and cardiovascular disease is not clear. In the most elementary terms, high blood pressure "tears up" the blood vessels in the body. A look at the conjunctiva reveals narrow and tortuous blood vessels (553),(570). Protein loss from the vasculature is greater than normal (744),(943).

Cardiovascular failure is a statistical process, with widely varying individual lifespans occurring at any given level of arterial pressure. Epidemiological studies (252),(421),(940) have identified a set of factors which increase an individual's risk of incurring cardiovascular disease. Besides high blood pressure, these include: obesity, smoking, diabetes and high serum cholesterol. For instance, Dyer (252) studied workers in Chicago and calculated big differences in predicted mortality rates over 14 years as a function of age, systolic blood pressure, serum cholesterol, and smoking habits.

PREDICTED MORTALITY OVER 14 YEARS

Age (Yrs)	Serum Cholesterol (mg/dl)	Systolic Pressure (mmHg)	Cigarettes (per day)	Mortality (%)
40	200	120	0	3
40	300	160	25	18
50	200	120	0	8
50	300	160	25	38

THE BENEFITS OF ANTIHYPERTENSIVE THERAPY

When blood pressure decreases, morbidity and mortality also decrease. This has been demonstrated in severe hypertension where death is imminent if treatment is not promptly instituted (573). It has been more difficult to conclusively demonstrate the decreased pressure - decreased morbidity relationship in those with mild essential hypertension. The results of recent clinical studies have been very persuasive, however. These data have provided the rationale for more aggressive treatment of hypertensive subjects who, because of a lack of acute discomfort, tend to ignore the opportunities offered by antihypertensive therapy.

The Veterans Administration study (960),(961),(962) demonstrated reductions in death, myocardial infarction, stroke, and heart failure with an adequate lowering of blood pressure. As an example, subjects with diastolic pressures between 90 mmHg and 114 mmHg were followed for an average of 3 to 4 years. Half received antihypertensive medication and half remained untreated. The treated group showed about four-tenths the mortality and one-fourth the morbidity of the untreated group (961) as summarized below.

BENEFITS OF ANTIHYPERTENSIVE THERAPY

	Untreated	Treated
Initial Arterial Pressure (mmHg)	165/105	162/104
Pressure After 4 Months	169/106	135/87
Number of Subjects	194	186
Total Morbid Events	35	9
Mortalities	19	8

ANTIHYPERTENSIVE DRUGS

Several different approaches have been evaluated in attempts to lower blood pressure. Manipulation of dietary salt intake was described in a previous chapter. Psychological methods have also been mentioned very briefly. To date, the major and most successful therapeutic approach has used drugs. Efficacy, pharmacology, specific applications, and side effects have been widely discussed in the clinical literature. The diversity of drugs currently available can be roughly grouped into: diuretics, beta-adrenergic blockers, sympatholytics, and direct vasodilators. These four groups will be discussed in the following sections with an interest in how their actions relate to the physiology of blood pressure control.

Diuretics

Although the terms "saluretic" and "natriuretic" are sometimes employed, the term "diuretic" is usually used to refer to drugs that produce both diuresis and natriuresis. The first diuretics were mercury compounds that had limited clinical value. Then, the observation of Schwartz (842) that sulfanilamide increased salt and water excretion in patients with heart failure prompted a methodical search for sulfanilamide-like compounds with diuretic properties at Merck, Sharpe and Dohme (77). The result was the discovery of the benzothiadiazines, and particularly chlorothiazide. About a dozen variations have since been developed that promote salt and water loss and lower arterial pressure.

Benzothiadiazines primarily inhibit sodium reabsorption in the distal tubule of the kidney. There are other diuretics, notably furosemide and ethacrynic acid, whose primary site of action is the loop of Henle. These are accordingly called "loop diuretics." Loop diuretics are generally reserved for acute applications because their brief duration of action offsets the advantage of exceptional potency. On the other hand, the benzothiadiazines are most suitable for long-term use and their antihypertensive properties will be discussed in more detail.

Acutely, diuretics increase salt and water excretion. Over longer periods excretion will be equal to intake whether or not a diuretic is being taken. Acute natriuresis decreases the body's exchangeable sodium, extracellular fluid volume, and plasma volume (187),(950),(951),(991). Over the longer term, these quantities tend to return to normal levels (951) although small sustained decreases in extracellular fluid volume have been reported (917),(950). Possible changes in lean body mass and other aspects of body composition over a prolonged period make interpretation difficult.

Arterial pressure falls gradually with diuretic administration. Cardiac output decreases acutely and then tends to increase slowly toward normal (187). The net result is a slowly developing vasodilation.

The way in which diuretics lower blood pressure is not understood. One explanation is that diuretics directly dilate the vasculature via mechanisms that are not related to changes in salt and water balance. One non-diuretic antihypertensive agent, diazoxide, has been shown to produce direct vasodilation and diazoxide's chemical structure is similar to many of the diuretics. But, the data in support of a direct vasodilator action for the diuretics is weak. Blood pressure falls slowly. And, it has recently been shown that furosemide has no acute effect on blood pressure in functionally anephric animals which should theoretically show all of the responses to diuretic administration except an enhanced salt and water excretion (648). It has also been proposed that diuretics will directly decrease vascular smooth muscle salt and water content, thereby producing vasodilation. Attempts to substantiate this have not succeeded, as reviewed by Tobian (933).

Salt and water loss from the body as a whole is an essential part of any diuretic-induced blood pressure decrease. The blood pressure decrease is prevented when enough salt is added to the diet to counterbalance the renal effects of the diuretic (991). This is consistent with the idea that reduced fluid volumes lead to reductions in cardiac output and these reductions in turn trigger autoregulatory vasodilation. The changes in cardiac output and peripheral resistance observed with diuretic administration give this explanation qualitative support. But, van Brummelen and colleagues have recently shown that transient decreases in cardiac output and plasma volume also occur in subjects who show no blood pressure decrease (949). Another idea is that sodium loss reduces the effectiveness of the sympathetic nervous system in producing vasoconstriction. None of these ideas is supported by compelling experimental evidence.

The blood pressure changes caused by diuretics are often much smaller than what would be expected for the amount of salt and water that is lost (360). The most likely explanation for this is that volume contraction stimulates renin release and the renin-angiotensin system in turn helps to maintain blood pressure at its original level (957). In experimental animals, volume contraction plus interruption of the renin-angiotensin system has been shown to cause dramatic decreases in arterial pressure in instances when volume contraction alone had little effect (344). Further, those patients who respond best to diuretic administration also show the smallest compensatory increase in plasma renin activity (548).

Diuretic administration enhances potassium excretion. Changes in the body's potassium stores probably do not play an important role in diuretic-induced blood pressure changes (991), but the resultant hypokalemia is a potentially serious side effect of long-term diuretic use (518).

Beta-adrenergic blockade

In 1948, Ahlquist (5) showed that there were two distinctly different types of catecholamine receptors in the body, and these have been called "alpha" and "beta" receptors. The alpha receptors are particularly sensitive to norepinephrine and generally produce vasoconstriction when stimulated. The beta receptors are particularly sensitive to isoproterenol and stimulation produces a variety of physiological effects including a strengthening of the heart, increased heart rate, vasodilation in some tissues, and renin release.

Several compounds resembling isoproterenol have been developed which bind to the beta-adrenergic receptors but do not stimulate them. Beta-adrenergic receptor blockers or beta-adrenergic antagonists are often called simply beta-blockers. These drugs have been widely used in quieting irregularities in heart rate and lowering blood pressure (770),(771). Excellent recent reviews have been provided by Tarazi and colleagues (916) and others (849),(179). At present, the most widely used beta-blocker is propranolol and many of the following citations refer to studies using this drug.

The way in which beta-blockers lower blood pressure is not known, and there is actually little reason to expect that they would lower blood pressure when known mechanisms of action are considered. Beta-blockade causes an immediate decrease in cardiac output (415),(944) that is apparently maintained indefinitely (32),(266),(329),(415),(608),(793). The fall in resting cardiac output is usually ascribed to decreased heart rate and myocardial contractility. Some decrease in the pumping ability of the heart is evident during exercise (767), but decreased cardiac function may not be the full explanation for low flow at rest since greater decreases in myocardial contractility can occur in myocardial infarction with far smaller changes in cardiac output. It may be that some aspect of oxygen uptake, delivery or metabolism is altered in such a way that lower blood flows are acceptable to the tissues (25). Oxygen consumption sometimes (117),(793), but not always (608), decreases with beta-blockade. Arteriovenous oxygen differences are increased (117). The oxygen dissociation characteristics of hemoglobin are altered (858). Before the hemodynamic actions of beta-blockade can be fully understood, it appears that more insight must be gained into the metabolic and autoregulatory properties of the tissues themselves.

Beta-blockade does not decrease vascular resistance (266),(415). Acutely, total peripheral resistance increases and it subsequently returns to near its original level with continuing blockade. Increased sympathetic nerve activity may be responsible for the initial vasoconstriction (663). Even though the numerical values do not indicate vasodilation, the eventual hemodynamic state might be considered to be a relative vasodilation in the sense that total peripheral resistance is lower during chronic beta-blockade than it would be in subjects having higher blood pressures and comparable cardiac outputs. Because of the persistent decrease in cardiac output, analyzing vascular resistance changes only in terms of the ratio of pressure to flow may obscure important underlying changes in regional circulatory function.

Beta-receptor blockade depresses renin secretion. When plasma renin activity is high, both renin levels and arterial pressure decrease in proportion with beta-blockade (126). In many instances, however, plasma renin activity is not particularly elevated in the first place, decreases are small, and a correlation between renin and pressure changes does not obtain (455),(649),(916). Beta-blockade has been shown to acutely depress renin secretion in salt-replete and salt-depleted subjects (898), but a much smaller chronic effect has been observed in sodium-depleted animals (888). Hence, renin suppression during beta-blockade may make some contribution to the overall antihypertensive effect but it does not appear to be a primary component.

Beta-blockers might lower blood pressure by decreasing sympathetic nerve activity, possibly acting on presynaptic receptors (4). Two studies (908),(581) have shown reduced sympathetic nerve activity after chronic treatment with propranolol and decreased adrenal catecholamine synthesis has also been observed (1). This is an attractive explanation for a phenomenon that has stubbornly resisted elucidation, but it is insufficiently developed at the present time.

Beta-blockade also has an effect on the central nervous system that becomes evident at high doses (179). It is not clear whether or not a central effect is an important component in the hypotensive response to beta-blockade.

Sympatholytics

A wide variety of drugs have been developed that interfere with sympathetic nervous function. Among the first were drugs which deplete peripheral norepinephrine stores or prevent norepinephrine release. Included in this category are the rauwolfia alkaloids, reserpine and guanethidine. Another early compound was hexamethonium, which interrupts sympathetic nerve traffic at the ganglia. Drugs were subsequently developed which bind to peripheral alpha-adrenergic receptors without stimulating them. These peripheral blockers include phentolamine and phenoxybenzamine. Monamine oxidase inhibitors decrease sympathetic activity, but the mechanisms involved are not clear. Of most recent interest are drugs which act on the central nervous system to decrease sympathetic outflow. Included in this category are clonidine and alpha-methyldopa.

All of the sympatholytics decrease sympathetic outflow or its effectiveness, leading to vasodilation in the peripheral vasculature and a decrease in arterial pressure. Some improvement in renal function may also be needed to offset the deliterious effects of falling blood pressure on renal excretion. It is sometimes observed that sympatholytics produce a rapid decrease in arterial pressure that is followed over the longer term by fluid retention and an apparent loss of efficacy (294),(386). Diuretics are beneficial in such instances.

One of the major complications arising from the aggressive use of sympatholytics is that the responsiveness of the baroreceptor reflexes is blunted. Upright posture without baroreceptor reflex compensation often leads to a severe hypotension that is not well tolerated.

Direct vasodilators

Compounds have been developed which directly suppress the contractility of vascular smooth muscle causing vasodilation. Included among these are hydralazine, guancydine, prazocin, diazoxide, and minoxidil. These drugs are known for their potency in that they literally force open blood vessels that had remained vasoconstricted with other antihypertensive therapy. Most of the citations below refer to studies using minoxidil.

The direct effect of these vasodilators on total peripheral resistance appears to be a straightforward phenomena. Minoxidil has been shown to produce decreased vascular resistance, decreased arterial pressure, and increased cardiac output (122). The persistent increase in cardiac output (122),(986) and muscle blood flow (19) suggests that either the metabolic needs of the body have been increased by this drug or, more likely, the drug is powerful enough to override the mechanisms that normally control blood flow.

Acutely, vasodilators produce tachycardia (465). This might be part of the baroreceptor response to a rapid decrease in arterial pressure. A Bainbridge response -- increased heart rate caused by increased ventricular filling -- has also been implicated. The tachycardia with minoxidil is persistent rather than transient and the reason for this is not known. Beta-blockade is often prescribed with minoxidil to prevent dangerously high heart rates from occurring.

Vasodilators should also affect the renal vasculature as they do other tissues, with renal vasodilation leading to an increase in renal function. However, fluid retention has been reported with the use of vasodilators in many instances and the concomitant administration of a diuretic is recommended. The cause of frequent fluid retention with direct vasodilation is not known, but renal vasodilation is probably not enough to offset the dramatic initial decrease in arterial pressure produced by vasodilation in other vascular beds. This would be likely if the vasodilator had a preferential effect on tissues other than the kidney (465),(798). This would also be likely in cases of advanced renal disease wherein little further improvement in renal function is possible. In total, direct vasodilators have proved to be a most useful antihypertensive approach, particularly in patients who are refractory to more conventional therapy and particularly when combined with a beta-adrenergic antagonist and diuretic. The use of direct vasodilators has also posed some very interesting physiological questions that have not yet been fully clarified.

CHAPTER 19

THE EFFECTS OF CONVERTING ENZYME INHIBITION

Several compounds have been discovered or created that inhibit angiotensin converting enzyme and thereby dramatically slow the conversion of angiotensin I to angiotensin II. One of these, captopril, has been widely used as an experimental tool and is currently being evaluated for routine clinical use because it can be administered orally.

Acute inhibition of angiotensin formation produces large decreases in blood pressure only when plasma renin activiity is grossly elevated, as in malignant hypertension or salt deprivation; in other instances acute inhibition has only a small hypotensive effect. With continuing or chronic inhibition, on the other hand, the acute effect is supplemented with a further, progressive decline in arterial pressure. Chronic treatment with captopril has been shown to lower blood pressure in hypertensions not associated with high levels of plasma renin, such as essential hypertension in humans and genetic hypertension in the Okamoto strain of rats. The cause of this potent antihypertensive effect is not clear. It has been postulated that bradykinin is responsible; converting enzyme is an enzyme that also controls bradykinin degradation and converting enzyme inhibition might lead to important increases in bradykinin levels. A renal factor may also be important, since inhibition often produces natriuresis and since arterial pressure falls gradually with chronic treatment as if a slow, cumulative process was at work. Acute studies have shown that converting enzyme inhibition increases renal blood flow, increases (but sometimes decreases) glomerular filtration rate, increases salt and water excretion and stimulates renin release. Diuretics in general have been observed to stimulate renin release and the renin in turn appears to blunt the antihypertensive effectiveness of the diuretic. Converting enzyme inhibition, in addition to providing a diuresis, will prevent the additional renin from being translated into more angiotensin II. Therefore, chronic inhibition might lower pressure via diuresis but without the hinderance usually produced by compensatory renin release.

The function of the renin-angiotensin system can also be interrupted using analogs of angiotensin II. Substitution of amino acids at the ends of the octapeptide sequence has produced variations of angiotensin with affinity for the angiotensin receptor but with attenuated activity. Use of these analogs has produced results that are qualitatively very similar to the results of converting enzyme inhibition. Synthesis of angiotensin analogs preceded the development of converting enzyme inhibitors; however, the use of analogs has been overshadowed by converting enzyme inhibition because analogs must be continuously infused to produce effective blockade and are not orally active.

THE RENIN-ANGIOTENSIN SYSTEM

Renin is an enzyme with a molecular weight of slightly greater than 40,000. It is synthetized primarily in the kidney and released into the circulating blood. Larger and less active proteins, called big renin and inactive renin, have been described and these may be the precursors of the active enzyme. Renin releases angiotensin I from a circulating alpha-2-globulin called renin substrate or angiotensinogen.

Angiotensin I is a decapeptide with the structure Asp-Arg-Val-Tyr-Ile- His-Pro-Phe-His-Leu. Angiotensin I has minimal biological activity. Angiotensin II is a biologically active decapeptide that is formed when angiotensin converting enzyme splits the carboxy-terminal histidylleucine (His-Leu) from angiotensin I. The structure and activity of angiotensin varies among the biological genera. A phylogenic review has been presented by Khosla and colleagues (510).

Angiotensin converting enzyme is actually one or more non-specific dipeptide carboxypeptidases found in the circulation and particularly in the lungs. Therefore, this enzyme also inactivates bradykinin by cleaving carboxy-terminal dipeptides. Bradykinin is a nonapeptide with the structure Arg-Pro-Pro-Gly-Phe-Ser-Pro-Phe-Arg.

There are several ways to interfere with the formation and action of angiotensin (623).

1. Decrease the activity of renin. Phospholipid inhibitors decrease the release and activity of renin. Pepstatin, a pentapeptide, decreases renin's enzymatic

activity (383), but it is most active at non-physiological pH's.

2. Use antibodies to bind renin or angiotensin. A variety of antibodies have been generated and used in physiological studies, but interpretation of results has been complicated by insufficient information about the titer and specificity of the antibodies used.

3. Occupy angiotensin receptors with inactive analogs of angiotensin. In 1970, Khairallah and colleagues (508) replaced phenylalanine with alanine at the 8 position on the angiotensin II molecule. The resulting peptide would bind to the angiotensin receptor without stimulating it. A search for angiotensin analogs showing minimal agonistic action, tight receptor binding, and slow metabolism followed.

4. Suppress angiotensin converting enzyme. Normally, the rate-limiting step in angiotensin II generation is provided by the enzyme renin rather than angiotensin converting enzyme. But, angiotensin II production falls to very low levels when converting enzyme is effectively inactivated. Of these different possibilities, angiotensin analogs and converting enzyme inhibitors have received the most attention.

EARLY CONVERTING ENZYME INHIBITORS

Converting enzyme inhibitors were first known as bradykinin potentiating peptides or bradykinin potentiating factors for their ability to depress the rate of metabolism of bradykinin within the body. Death by snake bite involves hypotension and this in turn could be due in part to excessive levels of bradykinin. As reported in 1965 from Ribeirao Preto, Brazil, substances in venom from the viper *Bothrops jararaca* enhance the effect of added bradykinin (281). Shortly thereafter it was shown that the lungs were the principal site for both bradykinin metabolism (284) and conversion of angiotensin I to angiotensin II (692). The action of a single enzyme was suspected, and this idea gained credance when Ferreira and colleagues (283) reported that a fraction of *Bothrops jararaca* venom decreased both bradykinin metabolism *and* angiotensin conversion.

Bothrops jararaca venom was subsequently shown to contain nine peptides containing from 5-13 amino acids (282). The pentapeptide, pyrrolidone carboxyl-Lys-Trp-Ala-Pro was sequenced (282), synthesized (895) and named Bradykinin Potentiating Peptide 5-alpha. BPP 5-alpha was shown by

Krieger and colleagues (542) to lower blood pressure, particularly when renin was suspected to be high.

It was subsequently shown that many different peptides will inhibit converting enzyme (717). These peptides have a wide range of biological half lives and affinities for converting enzyme. All are inactivated fairly rapidly. Of all the peptides first synthesized by Ondetti and colleagues (717), the nonapeptide pyrrolidone carboxyl-Trp-Pro-Arg-Pro-Gln-Ile-Pro-Pro appeared to most promising (46). This substance was first known as SQ 20,881 and then teprotide. Uncountable studies beginning in the early 1970's have used this substance to study the activity of the renin-angiotensin system and its possible role in the genesis of hypertension. Teprotide could not be given orally.

In 1977, Ondetti and colleagues (716) announced the development of an orally active converting enzyme inhibitor with the structure: D-3-mercapto-2-methylpropanoyl -L-proline. This substance was first known as SQ 14,225 and it is now called captopril. Captopril opened new horizons in blood pressure research because oral administration allowed chronic blockade of angiotensin II formation. Possible therapeutic value was considered from the start and captopril is currently undergoing evaluation as an antihypertensive drug.

ANGIOTENSIN ANALOGS vs CONVERTING ENZYME INHIBITORS

An alternative method for removing the effects of endogenous angiotensin II involves the use of angiotensin analogs. A variety of peptides have been configured that bind to angiotensin II receptors without producing the full effect of the naturally occurring molecule. These peptides are classified an angiotensin II antagonists with the most popular being 1-Sar, 8-Ala angiotensin II (738) and 1-Sar, 8-Ile angiotensin II (509). This nomenclature means that sarcosine has been substituted for aspartic acid at the 1 location on the molecule while alanine or isoleucine has been substituted for phenylalanine at the 8 location. Successful antagonists must bind tightly to the angiotensin receptor, have little agonistic effect, and be resistant to rapid metabolism. It appears that the amino acid at the 1 location determines strength of binding and rate of metabolism while the 8 location strongly influences biological activity (127),(787). Angiotensin

analogs are generally administered by the intravenous route. Because of rapid metabolism, a constant infusion is usually employed to insure steady occupancy of the angiotensin receptors by the analog.

There are many similarities in the biological responses to converting enzyme inhibition and angiotensin analog. In both cases a rapid decrease in arterial pressure is observed that is roughly proportional to the prevailing plasma renin activity. Converting enzyme inhibition in general shows greater depressor responses than the angiotensin analogs currently in use. These differences may be due to an inherent angiotensin-like (agonistic) action of the analog which diminishes the hypotensive responses and/or they may be due to an additional vasodepressor action of converting enzyme inhibitor. Some insight can be gained from protocols that directly compare the pressure decreases produced by these two agents (185),(186),(310). Regressions show that a pressure increase can be expected with angiotensin analogs when plasma renin activity is low; this demonstrates an inherent agonistic or pressor effect. Conversely, regressions show that no change in pressure or a decrease can be expected with converting enzyme inhibition when plasma renin activity is low; this implicates a non-renin, vasodepressor effect. The difference between the two responses in roughly 10 to 20 mmHg. Using a slightly different approach, it has sometimes (621),(929) but not invariably (479) been shown that converting enzyme inhibitor produces a further decrease in arterial pressure when given after angiotensin analog.

Davis and colleagues (214) have reviewed the use of angiotensin analogs to 1974. Because the analogs must be administered continuously and cannot be given orally, most recent activity has focused on the orally-active converting enzyme inhibitor, captopril. These results will be highlighted.

THE HEMODYNAMIC EFFECTS OF CONVERTING ENZYME INHIBITION

Many of the early studies using converting enzyme inhibition and angiotensin analogs focused on the acute blood pressure response to administration of these agents. Arterial pressure falls sharply and the size of the decrease has been shown to be rougly proportional to the level of plasma renin activity before inhibition. Plasma renin activity and plasma angiotensin I rise after converting enzyme inhibition (629).

Longer-term studies have shown that the blood pressure decrease with chronic administration can be considerably greater than the acute decreases. Laragh and colleagues (140), (561) have demonstrated a triphasic pattern in which the first phase is the acute fall in blood pressure just described. This is followed by no further decrease in pressure and in most instances a recovery of blood pressure toward normal. When inhibition is continued for periods of longer than a few days, there is a third phase to the response which includes a continuing decrease in blood pressure to even lower levels. The cause of these time-dependent effects is not clear but it can be postulated that the initial decrease is due to a removal of the direct vasoconstrictor effects of circulating angiotensin II. This is probably followed by compensations which tend to maintain or raise pressure; such compensations could include increased sympathetic activity, fluid shifts from the cells and interstitium into the circulation, further increases in plasma angiotensin I that would tend to override the effect of decreased converting enzyme activity, or other currently unsuspected compensations. The long-term, further decrease in blood pressure might be connected with an improvement in salt and water excretion, resetting of the baroreceptors, a function of bradykinin, or something else.

Anephric subjects

After the kidneys are removed, angiotensin analogs produce a moderate increase in pressure and this can be thought of as the antagonist activity of the analogs being displayed without the normal depressor contributions from antagonism of endogenous angiotensin II.

Several reports have indicated that converting enzyme inhibition produces little or no decrease in arterial pressure after the kidneys are removed (479),(576),(621). These data support the idea that inhibition produces a fast decrease in blood pressure when the kidneys are in by stopping the formation of angiotensin II and removing its direct vasoconstrictor effect on vascular smooth muscle. But this explanation may be too simple. Recent studies by Man in't Veld and colleagues (613) have shown that converting enzyme inhibition in hemodialysis patients without kidneys can cause a remarkable fall in arterial pressure. Subjects that are normally hydrated show the usual minimal response to converting enzyme inhibition. In contrast, subjects that have been volume depleted by ultrafiltration show a marked hypotensive response to converting enzyme inhibition even when there is little or no endogenous angiotensin II formation to be interfered with. The observed hypotensive response may be due to the formation of excess bradykinin, but there is little evidence to support this idea at the present time.

Normal subjects

When humans or experimental animals on a normal sodium intake are given converting enzyme inhibitor, arterial pressure falls from 0 to 10 mmHg (63),(479). Chronic administration roughly doubles this response to a pressure decrease of 10 to 20 mmHg (63). Chronic administration is sometimes accompanied by increased sodium excretion (63).

The simplest interpretation of this data is that the renin-angiotensin system supports up to 10mmHg of arterial pressure by direct vasoconstriction and up to 20 mmHg by direct vasoconstriction plus other longer-term mechanisms. The longer-term mechanisms may be related to salt and water balance. Administered angiotensin has been shown to be antinatriuretic. Conversely, elimination of endogenous angiotensin might be natriuretic. This phenomenon would take some time to develop -- just as the hypotensive action of diuretics is not immediately apparent.

Salt-depleted subjects

Sodium restriction using a low-salt diet or sodium depletion using the same diet plus administration of natriuretic drugs reduces the exchangeable sodium and extracellular fluid volume within the body. Plasma renin activity increases to up to ten times the normal, salt-replete level. However, arterial pressure shows little change during these protocols and both small increases and small decreases in pressure have been reported. Converting enzyme inhibition during salt restriction or depletion causes a marked, rapid, and continuing decrease in arterial pressure (63),(406),(407). Arterial pressures from 60 to 80 mmHg are commonly observed. Sodium excretion increases in these circumstances (63),(407), but the net sodium loss is probably too small to have a significant effect on arterial pressure. The data in total demonstrate that the renin-angiotensin system plays a very important role in maintaining arterial pressure when the salt and water stores of the body have fallen below normal.

Hypertensive subjects

Acute administration of converting enzyme inhibitor lowers blood pressure in hypertensive subjects and chronic administration produces even greater decreases (106), (119), (486). The magnitude of the blood pressure decrease is often proportional to the prevailng plasma renin activity (119), (140). Plasma renin activity is unmeasurably low in hypertension due to mineralocorticoid excess; converting enzyme inhibition causes little (239),(621) or no (243) decrease in arterial pressure. In contrast, large decreases in blood pressure have been reported when prevailing plasma renin activity is high such as in severe or malignant renal hypertension (118) or with concomitant sodium depletion (106), (486).

The total response to chronic converting enzyme inhibition is determined by more than the prevailing plasma renin activity. A significant correlation between the long-term blood pressure decrease and initial plasma renin activity does not always obtain in clinical studies (343). Animal studies may provide some insight. The data in general indicate that long-term converting enzyme inhibition causes big decreases in blood pressure in the two-kidney Goldblatt model (23),(62),(317), (796),(810) but only minor decreases in the one-kidney Goldblatt model (62). Inhibition will slow (317),(653),(975) but will not prevent (975) the onset of one-kidney hypertension.

Bengis and Coleman (62) showed that chronic inhibition would lower blood pressure all the way to normal in animals made hypertensive by renal artery stenosis with the contralateal kidney left untouched. In animals prepared with a comparable renal artery stenosis but contralateral nephrectomy, chronic inhibition lowered pressure approximately the same amount as seen in normal animals and normotension was not attained. This data is summarized on the next page.

BLOOD PRESSURE (mmHg) DURING CHRONIC INHIBITION OF CONVERTING ENZYME (62),(63)

	Control Pressure	Lowest Pressure	PRA*
Normal Animals	98	87	1.1
Salt Depleted	98	74	8.5
Goldblatt Hypertension:			
Benign 1-Kidney	150	126	1.0
Malignant 1-Kidney	184	132	4.2
Benign 2-Kidney	131	95	2.3
Malignant 2-Kidney	181	95	8.6

* ng AI/ml/hr

Although the animals with intact contralateral kidneys tended to have higher levels of plasma renin activity, there was enough overlap in plasma renin activities between the two models to illustrate that animals with high plasma renin activity and clamp plus nephrectomy did not approach normotension while animals with lower plasma renin activity and clamp plus intact kidney rapidly approached normotensive levels of blood pressure with chronic converting enzyme inhibition. These differences have not yet been adequately explained but it has been postulated that converting enzyme inhibition improves the excretory function of the intact contralateral kidney in the two-kidney model in a way that tends to lower blood pressure; this result is not possible in the animal with clamp plus contralateral nephrectomy. In total, it appears that the hypotensive action of converting enzyme inhibitor depends on the prevailing levels of plasma renin activity and on additional factors which are less well understood.

Another example of an unusual response to converting enzyme inhibition can be found in the response of the spontaneously hypertensive rat. The Okomoto strain is generally thought to have unusually high activity of the sympathetic nervous system while studies of the renin-angiotensin system have shown activity that is essentially normal in all respects, as reviewed in a previous chapter. Yet, converting enzyme inhibition over a few weeks reduces arterial pressure or prevents further increases in pressure in Okamoto rats (198),(285),(519),(825). Some studies have shown that full normotension can be achieved. Converting enzyme inhibition for one month produced a mean arterial pressure of 107 mmHg while comparable untreated Okomoto spontaneously hypertensive rats registered a mean pressure of 165 mmHg (825). These examples of striking reductions in blood pressure do not seem to be directly related to plasma renin activity nor are they acute. At the present time, the reason for this slowly developing, very powerful hypotensive response to converting enzyme inhibition is not known.

The use of converting enzyme inhibitor, specifically captopril, to treat hypertension in humans is being evaluated at this time and many preliminary reports have become available. Captopril has been shown to be a potent antihypertensive agent in hypertensions with a renal basis and in essential hypertension (31),(119),(343),(486),(966). The feeling at this time is that the hypotensive response can be roughly correlated to the prevailing plasma renin activity, but many subjects with plasma renin activities close to normal have shown a satisfactory decrease in blood pressure with treatment. Captopril plus sodium restriction or diuretics appears to be very effective in stubborn cases (106), (159), (486).

CONVERTING ENZYME INHIBITION AND THE KIDNEY

Inhibition of the formation of angiotensin II causes changes in renal hemodynamics, filtration, and excretion. The response is heightened when sodium depletion is used to raise renin and angiotensin levels before inhibition. These effects are not unexpected since Hollenberg *et al* (452) and others (460) have shown that the renal vasculature is unusually sensitive to added angiotensin II; we would expect the cessation of angiotensin II formation to result in equally striking but opposite changes.

Renal blood flow increases as arterial pressure is decreasing with inhibition (45),(403),(406),(407),(454),(512),(690), illustrating that angiotensin is a potent renal vasoconstrictor. Changes in glomerular filtration rate are variable. Increased filtration with inhibition has been observed in animals (512) and in some hypertensive subjects (453); in other instances, filtration shows little change (403),(690) or even falls (45),(406),(407) during inhibition even though renal blood flow has increased. Filtration fraction, the ratio of glomerular filtration rate and renal plasma flow, is usually decreased in these protocols showing that the blood flow response to inhibition is greater than the filtration rate response.

Converting enzyme inhibition could selectively vasodilate the afferent renal vessels, selectively dilate the efferent vessels, or generally affect both. Afferent dilation would tend to increase renal blood flow and filtration in proportion. Efferent dilation would tend to increase renal blood flow while decreasing or maintaining glomerular filtration rate. Therefore, efferent dilation would explain those observations in which renal blood flow increases while filtration rate decreases; these considerations and other data (404),(481), (785) suggest that angiotensin can have a selective efferent effect. However, there are exceptions to this (690) and the precise reasons remain unclear.

Converting enzyme inhibition increases salt and water excretion even in the face of falling arterial pressure (403),(407),(512). Increased renal blood flow might help to promote natriuresis, but a contribution from increased filtration is out of the question in instances in which filtration remains unchanged or falls. Available evidence suggests that converting enzyme inhibition may be removing a direct effect of angiotensin on tubular sodium reabsorption (406),(417),(485).

The natriuretic response to converting enzyme inhibition could contribute to the overall antihypertensive properties of available inhibitors. While sodium balance with continuing administration of converting enzyme inhibitor is often only mildly negative, there is an important further consideration. Diuretics decrease the body's sodium stores, but the antihypertensive response is usually blunted by compensatory increases in plasma renin activity. Therefore, the full effect of small decreases in body sodium does not become apparent in these instances. In the case of converting enzyme inhibition, compensatory increases in plasma renin activity also occur but the inhibitor prevents additional vasoconstriction. This suggests that the natriuresis produced by converting enzyme inhibition, however small, might make a significant contribution to the inhibitors' total antihypertensive effect by augmenting the pressure decreases produced by direct vascular vasodilation.

CONVERTING ENZYME INHIBITION AND BRADYKININ

Converting enzyme also regulates the metabolism of bradykinin. Inhibition slows the metabolism of bradykinin and the possibility exists that increased blood levels of bradykinin will occur and will contribute to the observed hypotensive response. Infused or injected bradykinin has been used to demonstrate this concept; the depressor response to bradykinin is greater and more prolonged following converting enzyme inhibition (686),(687).

The effect of inhibition on endogenous bradykinin has been much more difficult to ascertain. Measurement of blood levels have shown that inhibition usually increases plasma bradykinin concentration, but the increases are not particularly large (17),(454),(464), (629),(905),(987). Anderson *et al* (17) found small increases in bradykinin with captopril but normal levels were not exceeded. The interesting observation was that the largest bradykinin increases were seen in those subjects that had the smallest hypotensive response to captopril administration. Swartz *et al* (905) found the opposite. The physiological importance of modest increases in plasma bradykinin is not known. Nevertheless, it is tempting to speculate that increases in bradykinin levels can augment the hypotensive response of converting enzyme inhibition.

CHAPTER 20

A SYNTHESIS OF THE ELEMENTS OF BLOOD PRESSURE CONTROL

Much is still to be learned about the control of blood pressure. Certain features have emerged, however, that distinguish short-term control from long-term control.

The short-term control of arterial pressure relies primarily on neural mechanisms. Baroreceptor reflexes originating in the carotid and aortic arteries have been known to exist for some time and are now extensively described. But, additional afferent pathways from the heart, lungs and other organs have been described; the exact function and quantitative importance of these neural pathways is not completely understood.

The long-term control of arterial pressure involves, at least, the kidneys. Supporting evidence comes from studying hypertension as an expression of inadequate pressure control and the observation that almost all forms of experimental hypertension involve some manipulation of the kidneys or imposed changes in kidney function. Further, the onset of hypertension is often accompanied by inadequate renal excretion and increased activity of the renin-angiotensin system. Renal depressor substances and renal-neural interactions may also be involved, but there is less evidence in support of these possibilities.

Long-term changes in arterial pressure are usually accompanied by changes in vascular resistance, with cardiac output remaining relatively fixed. A connection between the renal release of renin, the generation of angiotensin within the circulating blood, and subsequent vasoconstriction is easy to visualize and intuitively pleasing. It is much harder to visualize a connection between changes in renal excretion and vasoconstriction, particularly in instances when angiotensin concentrations are low such as anephric hypertension or mineralocorticoid excess. Several explanations have been offered, including a scheme of autoregulatory vasoconstriction following salt and water retention and a direct effect of excess sodium on vascular smooth muscle. Both of these explanations are underpinned by supporting evidence, but much of the evidence is too indirect to permit a firm conclusion.

Several complexities must be dealt with in analyzing blood pressure control. Firstly, interventions that involve the kidneys will probably influence both renal excretion of salt and water and renal secretion of renin. Changes may or may not be complimentary. Secondly, circulating vasoconstrictors will simultaneously affect both vascular smooth muscle and renal excretion. For instance, angiotensin in excess can cause an elevation in arterial pressure by direct vasoconstriction but it may also have a less direct influence on pressure by modifying renal fuction in an antinatriuretic way. The complex interaction of these factors and many additional components in the long-term control of blood pressure makes it desirable to separate the components and to identify the quantitative importance of each. That is, the dominant components must be distinguished from the less important. With the evidence and analyses available to date, a tentative conclusion is that renal excretion of salt and water, particularly modulated by the activity of the renin-angiotensin system, is a very important factor or the most important factor in blood pressure control over the long term.

Human hypertension illustrates a defect in the long-term control of arterial pressure. This hypertension is usually presented with few obvious physiological abnormalities and consequently an acceptable explanation of the cause of essential hypertension is not now available. If analogies can be drawn between human essential hypertension and the performance of a variety of experimental animal models, it seems plausible that a renal defect, possibly involving salt and water excretion, is responsible.

THEORETICAL ANALYSES OF BLOOD PRESSURE CONTROL

Mathematical expressions can be used to describe and analyze biological processes in a manner that is both qualitatively and quantitatively rigorous. The circulatory system is particularly amenable to such analysis because well characterized physical processes often underlie complex circulatory phenomena. Early mathematical models focused on very specific cardiovascular events using simple mathematical descriptions. The scope of such analyses was probably limited by the lack of suitable analytical tools. But, the advent of powerful digital and analog computers has made it posible for recent analyses to include the breath and detail demanded by the complexeties of general blood pressure control (163).

Valid analyses require more than just adequate detail, however. Biological processes, simple or complex, must be described that are powerful enough to maintain pressure within normal limits during full range of simulated external and internal disturbances -- just as in reality.

Many models have concentrated on detailed anatomical descriptions or regional hemodynamic events (164). For instance, several early models such as the Windkessel model (697) were concerned with the genesis and propagation of pressure pulsations within the arteries. Such models are generally more relevant to isolated and specific physiological concepts than to overall blood pressure control.

In 1959 Grodins (376) published a mathematical analysis of short-term arterial pressure control. Guyton and colleagues subsequently developed several mathematical models (389),(391),(392),(393),(394), beginning in 1967, describing both the long- and short-term components of blood pressure control. These models have focused on the role of renal salt and water excretion in pressure control and on autoregulation as a possible cause of vasoconstriction in hypertension. Other simular analyses have investigated pressure control in general (229),(470) or during special situations such as established hypertension (145), changes in posture (102), hemodialysis (165), or the stresses of acceleration (34). Other circulatory models have been primarily didactic (483),(807),(931).

Mathematical analyses could contribute to blood pressure research (161). by fostering unambiguous thinking and stimulating hypothesis building and testing that is consonant with rigorous scientific method (163). While these are commendable uses, it should be noted that misuses are also possible (71). Generally, complex processes do not lend themselves well to verbal analysis; mathematical approaches may offer a novel adjunct to traditional laboratory and clinical studies of blood pressure control.

Unfortunately, mathematical analyses and the accompanying documentation seldom obtain a form that lends itself to easy publication via conventional channels. An uncertain number of models, such as those used by the National

Aeronautics and Space Administration, remain relatively uncirculated and unknown to most of the scientific community.

REFERENCES

1. Ablad B, Almgren A, Carlsson A, Henning M, Jonasson J, Ljung B. Reduced adrenal amine synthesis in spontaneously hypertensive rats after long-term treatment with propranolol. Brit J Pharmacol 61: 318-320, 1977.

2. Abramson DI, Fierst SM. Resting blood flow and peripheral vascular responses in hypertensive subjects. Amer Heart J 23: 84-96, 1942.

3. Addison W. The uses of sodium chloride, potassium chloride, sodium bromide and potassium bromide in cases of arterial hypertension which are amenable to potassium chloride. Canad Med Ass J 18: 281-285, 1928.

4. Adler-Graschinsky E, Langer S. Possible role of a beta-adrenoceptor in the regulation of noradrenaline release by nerve stimulation through a positive feed-back mechanism. Brit J Pharmacol 53: 43, 1975.

5. Ahlquist RP. A study of the adrenotropic receptors. Amer J Physiol 153: 586-600, 1948.

6. Albrecht I, Hallback M, Julius S, Lundgren Y, Stage L, Weiss L, Folkow B. Arterial pressure, cardiac output and systemic resistance before and after pithing in normotensive and spontaneously hypertensive rats. Acta Physiol Scand 94: 378-385, 1975.

7. Alexander JK. Obesity and the circulation. Mod Conc Cardiovas Dis 32: 799-803, 1963.

8. Alexander N, DeQuattro V. Regional and systemic hemodynamic patterns in rabbits with neurogenic hypertension. Circ Res 35: 636-645, 1975.

9. Alexander N, Heptinstall RH, Pickering GW. The effects of embolic obstruction of intrarenal arteries in the rabbit. J Pathol Bacteriol 81: 225-237, 1961.

10. Alexander N, Velasquez MT, Decuir M, Maronde RF. Indices of sympathetic activity in the sinoaortic-denervated hypertensive rat. Amer J

Physiol 238: H521-H526, 1980.

11. Alexander NL, Hinshaw B, Drury DR. Development of a strain of spontaneously hypertensive rabbits. Proc Soc Exp Biol Med 86: 855-858, 1954.

12. Allen FM, Scharf R, Lundin H. Clinical and experimental renal deficiency. JAMA 85: 1698-1701, 1925.

13. Alpert BS, Bain HH, Balfe JW, Kidd BSL, Olley PM. Role of the renin- angiotensin-aldosterone system in hypertensive children with coarctation of the aorta. Amer J Cardiol 43: 828-834, 1979.

14. Altman PL, Dittmer DS (Eds). Respiration and Circulation. Federation of American Societies for Experimental Biology, Bethesda, MD, 1971, pp. 399-413.

15. Amery A, Strooband R, Fagard R. Prognosis in low renin hypertension. New Eng J Med 288: 267, 1973.

16. Ames RP, Borkowski AJ, Sicinski AM, Laragh JH. Prolonged infusions of angiotensin II and norepinephrine on blood pressure, electrolyte balance and aldosterone and cortisol secretion in normal man and in cirrhosis of the liver. J Clin Invest 44: 1171-1186, 1965.

17. Anderson GH Jr, Springer J, Tivnan E, Kearney M, Streeten DHP. Hypotensive mechanism of captopril. Clin Res 28: 328A, 1980.

18. Anderson WP, Casley DJ. Role of the autonomic nervous system in the acute response to renal artery pressure reduction in conscious dogs. Clin Exp Pharmacol Physiol 7: 311-318, 1980.

19. Andersson O, Sivertsson R. Renal function and vascular resistance during long-term minoxidil treatment of severe hypertension. J Cardiovas Pharmacol 2(Suppl II): s123-s130, 1980.

20. Angell-James JE. Characteristics of single aortic and right subclavian baroreceptor fiber activity in rabbits with chronic renal hypertension. Circ Res 32: 149-161, 1973.

21. Annest JL, Sing CF, Biron P, Mongeau JG. Familial aggregation of blood pressure and weight in adoptive families. I. Comparisons of blood pressure and weight statistics among families with adopted, natural, or both natural and adopted children. Amer J Epidem 110: 479-491, 1979.

22. Annest JL, Sing CF, Biron P, Mongeau JG. Familial aggregation of blood pressure and weight in adoptive families. II. Estimation of the relative contributions of genetic and common environmental factors to blood pressure correlations between family members. Amer J Epidem 110: 492-503, 1979.

23. Antonaccio MJ, Rubin B, Horovitz ZP, Machaness G, Panasevich R. Long-term efficacy of captopril (SQ 14225) in two-kidney renal hypertensive rats. Clin Exp Hyperten 1: 505-519, 1979.

24. Aoki K, Yamori Y, Ooshima A, Okamoto K. Effects of high or low sodium intake in spontaneously hypertensive rats. Jap Circ J 36: 539-545, 1972.

25. Aoyagi M, Deshmukh VR, Meyer JS, Kawamura Y, Tagashira Y. Effect of beta-adrenergic blockade with propranolol on cerebral blood-flow, autoregulation and CO2 responsiveness. Stroke 7: 291-295, 1976.

26. Apfelbach CW, Jensen CR. Experimental chronic renal insufficiency in dogs, with special reference to arterial hypertension. J Clin Invest 10: 162-163, 1931.

27. Apfelbaum M, Boudon P, Lacatis D, Nillus P. Effets mataboliques de la diete protidique chez 41 sujets obese. Presse Med 78: 1917-1920, 1970.

28. Arendshorst WJ. Autoregulation of the renal blood flow in spontaneously hypertensive rats. Circ Res 44: 344-349, 1979.

29. Arrizurieta de Muchnik EE, Lipham EM, Gottschalk CW. Form and function in normal and hypertrophied nephrons. pp 29-42 in Compensatory Renal Hypertrophy eds WW Nowinski, RJ Gross. Academic Press, New York, 1969.

30. Arterial Hypertension. Technical Report Series, 628. World Health Organization, Geneva, 1978.

31. Atlas SA, Case DB, Sealey JE, Laragh JH, McKinstry DN. Interruption of the renin-angiotensin system in hypertensive patients by captopril induces sustained reduction in aldosterone secretion, potassium retention and natriuresis. Hypertension 1: 274-280, 1979.

32. Atterhog H, Duner H, Pernow B. Hemodynamic effect of pindolol in essential hypertension with special reference to the resistance and capacitance vessels of the forearm. Acta Med Scand 199: 251-255, 1976.

33. Aurell M, Pettersson M, Berglund G. Renin-angiotensin system in essential hypertension. Lancet 2: 342-345, 1975.

34. Avula XJR, Oestreicher HL. Mathematical model of the cardiovascular system under acceleration stress. Aviat Space Environ Med 49: 279-286, 1978.

35. Axelrod J, Cohn CK. Methyltransferase enzymes in red blood cells. J Pharmacol Exp Ther 176: 650-654, 1971.

36. Axelrod J, Tomchick R. Enzymatic O-methylation of epinephrine and other catechols. J Biol Chem 233: 702-705, 1958.

37. Ayers CR, Katholi RE, Vaughn ED Jr, Carey RM, Kimbrough HM Jr, Yancey MR, Morton CL. Intrarenal renin-angiotensin-sodium interdependent mechanism controlling postclamp renal artery pressure and renin release in the conscious dog with chronic one-kidney Goldblatt hypertension. Circ Res 40: 238-242, 1977.

38. Ayitey-Smith E, Varma DR. An assessment of the role of the sympathetic nervous system in experimental hypertension using normal and immunosympathectomised rats. Brit J Pharmacol 40: 175-185, 1970.

39. Ayman D, Goldshine AD. Blood pressure determinations by patients with essential hypertension. I. The difference between clinic and home readings before treatment. Amer J Med Sci 200: 465-474, 1940.

40. Azar S, Johnson MA, Scheinman J, Bruno L, Tobian L. Regulation of glomerular capillary pressure and filtration rate in young Kyoto hypertensive rats. Clin Sci 56: 203-209, 1979.

41. Baer PG, Bianchi G. Renal micropuncture study of normotensive and Milan hypertensive rats before and after development of hypertension. Kid Inter 13: 452-466, 1978.

42. Bagby SP, Mass RD. Abnormality of the renin/body-fluid-volume relationship in serially-studied inbred dogs with neonatally-induced coarctation hypertension. Hypertension 2: 631-642, 1980.

43. Bagby SP McDonald WJ, Mass RD. Serial renin-angiotensin studies in spontaneously hypertensive and Wistar-Kyoto normotensive rats. Hypertensive 1: 347-354, 1979.

44. Bagby SP, McDonald WJ, Strong DW, Porter GA, Bennet WM, Bonchek, LI. Abnormalities of renal perfusion and the renal pressor system in dogs with chronic aortic coarctation. Circ Res 37: 615-620, 1975.

45. Bailie MD, Barbour JA. Effect of inhibition of peptidase activity on distribution of intrarenal blood flow. Amer J Physiol 228: 850-853, 1975.

46. Bakhle YS. Inhibition of angiotensin I converting enzyme by venom peptides. Brit J Pharmacol 43: 252-254, 1971.

47. Balomey AA, Michie AJ, Michie C, Breed ES, Schreiner GE, Lauson HD. Simultaneous measurement of effective renal blood flow and cardiac output in resting normal subjects and patients with essential hypertension. J Clin Invest 28: 10-17, 1949.

48. Barajas L. The innervation of the juxtaglomerular apparatus. Lab Invest 13: 916-929, 1964.

49. Barajas L. Innervation of the renal cortex. Fed Proc 1192-1201, 1978.

50. Barsanti JA, Pillsbury HRC III, Freis ED. Enhanced salt toxicity in the spontaneously hypertensive rat. Proc Soc Exp Biol Med 136: 565-568, 1971.

51. Battarbee HD, Funch DP, Dailey JW. The effect of dietary sodium and potassium upon blood pressure and catecholamine excretion in the rat. Proc Soc Exp Biol Med 161: 32-37, 1979.

52. Bauer JH, Brooks CS. Volume studies in men with mild to moderate hypertension. Amer J Cardiol 44: 1163-1170, 1979.

53. Bauman L. Obesity. Recent reports in the literature and results of treatment. JAMA 90: 22-24, 1929.

54. Baxter JD, Schambelan M, Matulich DT, Spindler BJ, Taylor AA, Bartter FC. Aldosterone receptors and the evaluation of plasma mineralocorticoid activity in normal and hypertensive states. J Clin Invest 58: 579-589, 1976.

55. Beaglehole R, Salmond CE, Eyles EF. A longitudinal study of blood pressure in Polynesian children. Amer J Epidem 105: 87-89, 1977.

56. Beaglehole R, Salmond CE, Prior IAM. A family study of blood pressure in Polynesians. Inter J Epidem 4: 217-220, 1975.

57. Bean BL, Brown JJ, Casals-Stenzel J, Fraser R, Lever AF, Millar JA, Morton JJ, Petch B, Riegger AJG, Robertson JIS, Tree M. The relation of arterial pressure and plasma angiotensin II concentration. A change produced by prolonged infusion of angiotensin II in the conscious dog. Circ Res 44: 452-458, 1979.

58. Beevers DG, Morton JJ, Nelson CS, Padfield PL, Titterington M, Tree M. Angiotensin II in essential hypertension. Brit Med J 1: 415, 1977.

59. Beilin LJ, Wade DN. Vascular hyperreactivity with sodium loading and with deoxycorticosterone induced hypertension in the rat. Nature 227: 1141-1142, 1970.

60. Bell DR, Overbeck HW. Increased resistance and impaired maximal vasodilation in normotensive vascular beds of rats with coarctation hypertension. Hypertension 1: 78-85, 1979.

61. Benedict CR, Grahame-Smith DG, Fisher A. Sequential measurement of plasma catecholamines and dopamine-beta-hydroxylase in patients who have undergone corrective surgery for coarctation of the aorta. Clin Sci Molec Med 52: 19P-20P, 1977.

62. Bengis RG, Coleman TG. Antihypertensive effect of

prolonged blockade of angiotensin formation in benign and malignant, one- and two-kidney Goldblatt hypertensive rats. Clin Sci 57: 53-62, 1979.

63. Bengis RG, Coleman TG, Young DB, McCaa RE. Long-term blockade of angiotensin formation in various normotensive and hypertensive rat models using converting enzyme inhibitor (SQ 14225). Circ Res 43(Suppl I): 45-53, 1978.

64. Benson H, Shapiro D, Tursky B, Schwartz GE. Increased systolic blood pressure through operant conditioning techniques in patients with essential hypertension. Science 173: 740-741, 1971.

65. Berecek KH, Bohr DF. Whole body vascular reactivity during development of deoxycorticosterone acetate hypertension in the pig. Circ Res 42: 764-771, 1978.

66. Berecek KH, Stocker M, Gross F. Changes in renal vascular reactivity at various stages of deoxycorticosterone hypertension in rats. Circ Res 46: 619-624, 1980.

67. Berenson GS, Srinivasan SR, Radhakrishnamurthy B, Dalferes ER Jr, Foster T, Voors AW. A nonhuman primate model for diet induced hypertension. Circulation 56(Suppl II): 242, 1977.

68. Beretta-Piccoli C, Weidmann P, Kensch G, Grimin M, Meier A, Gluck Z, Ziegler WH. Renin-hyporesponsiveness in essential hypertension. Dissociation between plasma renin and carecholamines or aldosterone following furosemide. Klin Wschr 58: 457-465, 1980.

69. Berglund G, Aurell M, Wilhelmsen L. Renal function in normo- and hypertensive 50 year old males. Acta Med Scand 199: 25-32, 1976.

70. Berglund G, Wikstrand J, Wallentin I, Wilhelmsen L. Sodium excretion and sympathetic activity in relation to severity of hypertensive disease. Lancet 1: 324-328, 1976.

71. Berlinski D. _On Systems Analysis: An Essay Concerning the Limitations of Some Mathematical Methods in the Social, Political, and Biological Sciences_. The MIT Press, Cambridge, 1976.

72. Bevan AT, Honour AJ, Stott FH. Portable recorder for continuous arterial pressure measurement in man. J Physiol 186: 3P, 1966.

73. Bevan AT, Honour AJ, Stott FH. Direct arterial pressure recording in unrestricted man. Clin Sci 36: 329-344, 1969.

74. Bevan JA, Bevan RD, Chang PC, Pegram BL, Purdy RE, Su C. Changes in the contractile response of arteries and veins from hypertensive rabbits to sympathetic nerve activity: Assessment of some post synaptic influences. Blood Vessels 13: 167-180, 1976.

75. Bevan RD, Eggena P, Hume WR, Loes LT, Van Marthens E, Bevan JA. An 8 month longitudinal study of changes in elastic and muscular arteries and veins of the rabbit with sustained hypertension after abdominal aorta constriction. Clin Sci 57: 7s-9s, 1979.

76. Bevan RD, Purdy RE, Su C, Bevan JA. Evidence for an increase in adrenergic nerve function in blood vessels from experimental hypertensive rabbits. Circ Res 37: 503-508, 1975.

77. Beyer KH Jr. Discovery of the thiazides: where biology and chemistry meet. Perspect Biol 20: 410-420, 1977.

78. Bianchi G, Baer PG, Fox U, Duzzi L, Caravaggi AM, Mohring J, Cusi D. Kidney function studies in the Milan hypertensive strain of rats. pp 144-151 in _The Kidney in Arterial Hypertension_, eds G Bianchi, G Bazzato. Bunge Scientific Publishers, Utrecht, 1979.

79. Bianchi G, Baer PG, Fox U, Duzzi L, Pagetti D, Giovannetti AM. Changes in renin, water balance, and sodium balance during development of high blood pressure in genetically hypertensive rats. Circ Res 36(Suppl I): 153-161, 1975.

80. Bianchi G, Baer PG, Fox U, Guidi E. The role of the kidney in the rat with genetic hypertension. Postgrad Med J 53: 123-135, 1977.

81. Bianchi G, Baldoli E, Lucca R, Barbin P. Pathogenesis of arterial hypertension after constriction of the renal artery leaving the opposite kidney intact both in the anesthetized and in the conscious dog. Clin

Sci 42: 651-664, 1972.

82. Bianchi G, Cusi D, Gatti M, Lupi GP, Ferrari P, Barlassina C, Picotti GB, Bracchi G, Colombo G, Gori D, Veles O, Mazzei D. A renal abnormality as a possible cause of "essential" hypertension. Lancet 1: 173-177, 1979.

83. Bianchi G, Fox U, DiFrancesco GF, Bardi U, Radice M. The hypertensive role of the kidney in spontaneously hypertensive rats. Clin Sci. Molec Med 45(Suppl):135s-139s, 1973.

84. Bianchi G, Fox U, DiFrancesco GF, Giovanetti AM, Pagetti D. Blood pressure changes produced by kidney cross-transplantation between spontaneously hypertensive rats and normotensive rats. Clin Sci Molec Med 47: 435-448, 1974.

85. Bianchi G, Fox U, Imbasciati E. The development of a new strain of spontaneously hypertensive rats. Life Sci 14: 339-347, 1974.

86. Bianchi G, Ponticelli C, Bardi V, Redaelli B, Campolo L, dePonti C, Graziani G. Role of the kidney in 'salt and water dependent hypertension' of end-stage renal disease. Clin Sci 42: 47-55, 1972.

87. Bianchi G, Tenconi LT, Lucca R. Effect in the conscious dog of constriction of the renal artery to a sole remaining kidney on the hemodynamics, sodium balance, body fluid volumes, plasma renin concentration and pressor responsiveness to angiotensin. Clin Sci 38: 741-766, 1970.

88. Biglieri EG, Forsham PH. Studies on the expanded extracellular fluid and the response to various stimuli in primary aldosteronism. Amer J Med 30: 564-576, 1961.

89. Bing RJ, Thomas CB, Waples EC. The circulation in experimental neurogenic hypertension. J Clin Invest 24: 513-522, 1945.

90. Birkenhager WH, Schalekamp MADH, Krauss XH, Kolsters G, Schalekamp-Kuyken MPA, Kroon BJM, Teulings FAG. Systemic and renal hemodynamics, body fluids and renin in benign essential hypertension with special reference to natural history. Europ J Clin Invest 2:

115-122, 1972.

91. Biron P, Mongeau JG, Bertrand D. The familial aggregation of blood pressure in childhood is hereditary. Pediatrics 54: 659-660, 1974.

92. Biron P, Mongeau JG, Bertrand D. Familial aggregation of blood pressure in 558 adopted children. Canad Med Ass J 115: 773-774, 1976.

93. Biron P, Mongeau JG, Bertrand D. Familial resemblance of body weight/height in 374 homes with adopted children. J Pediat 91: 555-558, 1977.

94. Blacket RB, Pickering GW, Wilson GM. The effects of prolonged infusions of noradrenaline and adrenaline on the arterial pressure of the rabbit. Clin Sci 9: 247-257, 1950.

95. Blair-West JR, Coghlon JP, Denton DA, Orchard E, Scoggins BA, Wright RD. Renin-angiotensin-aldosterone system and sodium balance in experimental renal hypertension. Endocrinology 83: 1199-1209, 1968.

96. Bohlen HG, Gore RW, Hutchins PM. Comparison of microvascular pressures in normal and spontaneously hypertensive rats. Microvas Res 13: 125-130, 1977.

97. Booth J. A short history of blood pressure measurement. Proc Roy Soc Med 70: 793-799, 1977.

98. Borst JGG, Borsr-de Geus A. Hypertension explained by Starling's theory of circulatory homoestasis. Lancet 1: 677, 1963.

99. Bounous G, Shumaker HB Jr. Experimental unilateral renal artery stenosis. Surg Gynec Obstet 114: 415-425, 1962.

100. Bower JD, Coleman TG. Circulatory function during hemodialysis. Trans Amer Soc Artif Intern Organs 15: 373-376, 1969.

101. Boyd JD, McCullagh GP. Experimental hypertension following carotico-aortic denervation in the rabbit. Quart J Exp Physiol 27: 293-306, 1938.

102. Boyers DG, Cuthbertson JG, Luetscher JA. Simulation of the human cardiovascular system: A model with

normal responses to change of posture, blood loss, transfusion, and autonomic blockade. Simulation 18: 197-206, 1972.

103. Bradford JR. The results following partial nephrectomy and the influence of the kidney upon metabolism. J Physiol 23: 415-496, 1898.

104. Braun-Menendez E. Hypophysis and blood pressure. Cardiologia 21: 272-283, 1952.

105. Braun-Menendez E, Fasciolo JC, Leloir LF, Munoz JM. The substance causing renal hypertension. J Physiol 89: 283-298, 1940.

106. Bravo EL, Tarazi RC. Converting enzyme inhibition with an orally active compound in hypertensive man. Hypertension 1: 39-46, 1979.

107. Bravo EL, Tarazi RC, Dustan HP. Mulifactorial analysis of chronic hypertension induced by electrolyte-active steroids in trained, unanesthetized dogs. Circ Res 40(Suppl I): 140-145, 1977.

108. Brod J. Essential hypertension: Hemodynamic observations with bearing on its pathogenesis. Lancet 2: 773-778, 1960.

109. Brod J. Hemodynamics and emotional stress. Bibl Psychiat 144: 13-33, 1970.

110. Brod J, Fencl V, Hejl Z, Sirka J, Ulrych M. General and regional haemodynamic pattern underlying essential hypertension. Clin Sci 23: 339-349, 1962.

111. Brody MJ, Fink GD, Buggy J, Haywood JR, Gordan FJ, Johnson AK. The role of the anteroventral third ventricle (AV3V) region in experimental hypertension. Circ Res 43(Suppl I): 2-13, 1978.

112. Brody MJ, Haywood JR, Touw KB. Neural mechanisms in hypertension. Ann Rev Physiol 42: 441-453, 1980.

113. Brown JJ, Chapuis G, Robertson JIS. The effect of long-continued intravenous infusions of angiotensin in the rabbit. Lancet 1: 1356-1357, 1963.

114. Brown JJ, Lever AF, Robertson JIS, Schalekamp MA.

Pathogenesis of essential hypertension. Lancet 1: 1217-1219, 1976.

115. Brown WJ Jr, Brown FK, Krishan I. Exchangable sodium and blood volume in normotensive and hypertensive humans on high and low sodium intake. Circulation 43: 508-519, 1971.

116. Brown WJ, Brown FK, Drishan I. Exchangeable sodium and blood volume in normotensive and hypertensive humans on high and low sodium intake. Circulation 43: 508-519, 1971.

117. Brundin T. Effects of beta-adrenergic receptor blockade on metabolic rate and mixed venous blood temperature during dynamic exercise. Scand J Clin Lab Invest 38: 229-232, 1978.

118. Brunner HR, Gavras H, Laragh JH, Keenan R. Angiotensin II blockade in man by Sar-1, Ala-8, angiotensin II for understanding and treatment of high blood pressure. Lancet 2: 1045-1048, 1973.

119. Brunner HR, Gavras H, Walker B, Kershaw GR, Turini GA, Vukovich RA, McKinstry DN, Gavras I. Oral angiotensin-converting enzyme inhibitor in long-term treatment of hypertensive patients. Ann Intern Med 90: 19-23, 1979.

120. Brunner HR, Kirshman JD, Sealey JE, Laragh JH. Hypertension of renal origin: Evidence for two different mechanisms. Science 174: 1344-1346, 1971.

121. Brunner HR, Laragh JH, Baer L, Newton MA, Goodwin FT, Krakoff LR, Buhler FR. Essential hypertension: renin and aldosterone, heart attack and stroke. New Eng J Med 286: 441-449, 1972.

122. Bryan RK, Hoobler SW, Rosenzweig J, Weller JM. Effect of minoxidil on blood pressure and hemodynamics in severe hypertension. Amer J Cardiol 39: 796-801, 1977.

123. Buggy J, Fink GD, Haywood JR, Johnson AK, Brody MJ. Interruption of the maintenance phase of established hypertension by ablation of the anteroventral third ventricle (AV3V) in rats. Clin Exp Hyperten 1: 337-353, 1978.

124. Buggy J, Fink GD, Johnson AK, Brody MJ. Prevention of the development of renal hypertension by anteroventral third ventricular tissue lesions. Circ Res 40(Suppl I): 110-117, 1977.

125. Buhler FR, Laragh JH, Sealey JE, Brunner HR. Plasma aldosterone-renin interrelationships in various forms of essential hypertension. Amer J Cardiol 32: 554-561, 1973.

126. Buhler FR, Laragh JH, Vaughan ED Jr, Brunner HR, Gavras H, Baer L. Antihypertensive action of propranolol. Amer J Cardiol 32: 511-522, 1973.

127. Bumpus FM, Sen S, Smeby RR, Sweet C, Ferrario CM, Khosla MC. Use of angiotensin II antagonists in experimental hypertension. Circ Res 32 (Suppl I): 150-158, 1973.

128. Bunag RD. Pressor effects of the tail-cuff method in awake normotensive and hypertensive rats. J Lab Clin Med 78: 675-682, 1971.

129. Burkhalter JF, Franklin SS, Maxwell MH, Lupu AN. Influence of posture and Na balance on plasma catecholamines in normal subjects, and in patients with essential and renovascular hypertension. Kid Inter 14: 692, 1978.

130. Butt TJ, Jones DR, Bolli P, Wallis AT, Simpson FO. Intrarenal blood flow distribution in the genetically hypertensive rat. Nephron 26: 49-52, 1980.

131. Byrom FB, Dodson LF. The mechanism of the vicious circle in chronic hypertension. Clin Sci 8: 1-10, 1949.

132. Byrom FB, Wilson C. A plethysmographic method for measuring systolic blood pressure in the intact rat. J Physiol 93: 301-304, 1938.

133. Caliva FS, Napodano RJ, Lyons RH. Digital hemodynamics in the normotensive and hypertensive states. II. Venomotor tone. Circulation 28: 421-426, 1963.

134. Cameron J, Meek AP, Phelan EL. Cardiac output of genetically hypertensive rats. New Zeal Med J 82: 389, 1975.

135. Campbell DJ, Skinner SL, Day AJ. Cellophane perinephritis hypertension and its reversal in rabbits. Circ Res 33: 105-112, 1973.

136. Caravaggi AM, Bianchi G, Brown JJ, Lever AF, Morton JJ , Powell-Jackson JD, Robertson JIS, Semple PF. Blood pressure and plasma angiotensin II concentration after renal artery constriction and angiotensin infusion in the dog. Circ Res 38: 315-321, 1976.

137. Carey RM, Dacey RG, Jane JA, Winn HR, Ayers CR, Tyson GW. Production of sustained hypertension by lesions in the nucleus tractus solitarii of the American foxhound. Hypertension 1: 246-254, 1979.

138. Carretero OA, Gulati OP. Effects of angiotensin antagonist in rats with acute, subacute, and chronic two-kidney renal hypertension. J Lab Clin Med 91: 264-271, 1978.

139. Carriere S. Influence of sodium intake on catecholamine release by renal nerve stimulation in dogs. Clin Res 26: 868A, 1978.

140. Case DB, Atlas SA, Laragh JH, Sullivan PA, Sealey JE. Use of first-dose response or plasma renin activity to predict the long-term effect of captopril: Identification of triphasic pattern of blood pressure response. J Cardiol Pharmacol 2: 339-346, 1980.

141. Chaireillo L, Agosti J, Subramanian S. Coarctation of the aorta in children and adolescents. Chest 70: 621-626, 1976.

142. Chalmers JB. Brain amines and models of experimental hypertension. Circ Res 36: 469-480, 1975.

143. Chanutin A, Ferris EB. Experimental renal insufficiency produced by partial nephrectomy. Arch Intern Med 49: 767-787, 1932.

144. Chapman CB, Gibbons TB. The diet and hypertension. Medicine 29: 29-60, 1950.

145. Chau NP, Safar ME, London GM, Weiss YA. Essential hypertension: An approch to clinical data by the use of models. Hypertension 1: 86-97, 1979.

146. Chau NP, Safar ME, Weiss YA, London GM, Simon AC, Milliez PL. The relationship between cardiac output, heart rate and blood volume in essential hypertension. Clin Sci Molec Med 54: 175-180, 1978.

147. Cheitlin MD. Coarctation of the aorta. Med Clin N Amer 61: 655-673, 1977.

148. Cherchovich GM, Capek K, Jefremova Z, Pohlova I, Jelinek J. High salt intake and blood pressure in lower primates (Papio hamadryas). J Appl Physiol 40: 601-604, 1976.

149. Chiang BN, Perlman LV, Epstein FH. Overweight and hypertension. Circulation 39: 403-421, 1969.

150. Chiueh CC, Kopin IJ. Hyperresponsivity of spontaneously hypertensive rat to indirect measurement of blood pressure. Amer J Physiol 234: H690-H695, 1978.

151. Chrysant SG, Walsh GM, Kern DC, Frohlich ED. Hemodynamic and metabolic evidence of salt sensitivity in spontaneously hypertensive rats. Kid Inter 15: 33-37, 1979.

152. Chrysanthakopoulos SG, Kastagir BK, Jubiz W, Kolff WJ. Hypertension in patients on maintenance hemodialysis: Evaluation of peripheral renin activity and bilateral nephrectomy. Amer J Med Sci 264: 9-21, 1972.

153. Clark DWJ. Effects of immunosypathectomy of development of high blood pressure in genetically hypertensive rats. Circ Res 28: 330-336, 1971.

154. Clark DWJ, Jones DR, Phelan EL, Devine CE. Blood pressure and vascular resistance in genetically hypertensive rats treated at birth with 6-hydroxydopamine. Circ Res 43: 293-300, 1978.

155. Clark DWJ, Phelan EL. Renal hypertension in rats chronically sympathectomized with 6-hydroxydopamine. Proc Univ Otago Med Sch 50: 44-46, 1972.

156. Clark DWJ, Phelan EL. Blood pressure and hindlimb perfusion pressure following chronic sympathectomy of genetically hypertensive and normotensive rats. Clin Exp Pharmacol Physiol (Suppl II): 153-157, 1975.

157. Clement DL. Blood Pressure Variability. University Park Press, Baltimore, 1979.

158. Coburn RJ, Manger WM, Dufton S, Gallo G, Manger CC III. Absence of renal participation in genesis of hypertension in spontaneously hypertensive rats (SHR). Clin Res 20: 589, 1972.

159. Cody RJ Jr, Tarazi RC, Bravo EL, Fouad FM. Hemodynamics of orally-active converting enzyme inhibitor (SQ 14225) in hypertensive patients. Clin Sci Molec Med 55: 453-459, 1978.

160. Cohen DM, Grekin RJ, Mitchell J, Rice WH, Bohr DF. Hemodynamic, endocrine and electrolyte changes during sodium restriction in DOCA hypertensive pigs. Hypertension 2: 490-496, 1980.

161. Coleman TG. Simulation is helping biomedical research. Simulation 19: 29-32, 1972.

162. Coleman TG. Cardiac output by dye dilution in the conscious rat. J Appl Physiol 37: 452-455, 1974.

163. Coleman TG. From Aristotle to modern computers: The role of theories in biological research. Physiologist 18: 509-518, 1975.

164. Coleman TG. Simulation of biological systems: The circulation of blood. Simulation 28: 201-204, 1977.

165. Coleman TG, Bower JD, Guyton AC. Chronic hemodialysis and circulatory function. Simulation 15: 222-228, 1970.

166. Coleman TG, Bower JD, Langford HG, Guyton AC. Regulation of arterial pressure in the anephric state. Circulation 42: 509-514, 1970.

167. Coleman TG, Granger HJ, Guyton AC. Whole-body circulatory autoregulation and hypertension. Circ Res 28(Suppl II): 76-87, 1971.

168. Coleman TG, Guyton AC. Hypertension caused by salt-loading: III. Onset transients of cardiac output and other circulatory parameters. Circ Res 25: 153-160, 1969.

169. Coleman TG, Guyton AC. The pressor role of

angiotensin in salt deprivation and renal hypertension. Clin Sci 48: 45s-48s, 1975.

170. Coleman TG, Guyton AC, Young DB, DeClue JW, Norman RA Jr, Manning RD Jr. The role of the kidney in essential hypertension. Clin Exp Pharmacol Physiol 2: 571-581, 1975.

171. Coleman TG, Manning RD Jr, Norman RA Jr, DeClue JW. The role of the kidney in spontaneous hypertension. Amer Heart J 89: 94-98, 1975.

172. Coleman TG, Samar RE, Murphy WR. Autoregulation versus other vasoconstrictors in hypertension. A critical review. Hypertension 1:324-330, 1979.

173. Collins DA. Hypertension from constriction of the arteries of denervated kidneys. Amer J Physiol 116: 616-621, 1936.

174. Collis MG, DeMey C, Vanhoutte PM. Renal vascular reactivity in the young spontaneously hypertensive rat. Hypertension 2: 45-52, 1980.

175. Collis MG, Vanhoutte PM. Vascular reactivity in the isolated perfused kidney of the spontaneously hypertensive rat. Arch Int Pharmacol 222: 164-165, 1976.

176. Comroe JH Jr. First annual Irving H. Page lecture : A Page in the story of hypertension. Cleveland Clin Quart 45: 311-323, 1978.

177. Conn JW. Presidential address. Part II. Primary aldosteronism, a new clinical syndrome. J Lab Clin Med 45: 6-17, 1955.

178. Conn JW. Primary aldosteronism. J Lab Clin Med 45: 661-664, 1955.

179. Conolly ME, Kersting F, Dollery CT. The clinical pharmacology of beta-adrenoceptor blocking drugs. Prog Cardiovas Dis 19: 203-234, 1976.

180. Conrad MC, Anderson JL III, Garrett JB. Chronic collateral growth after femoral artery occusion in the dog. J Appl Physiol 31: 550-555, 1971.

181. Conway FJ, Hatton R. The effects of

beta-adrenoceptor blockade on the development of deoxycorticosterone acetate hypertension in the dog. Brit J Pharmacol 60: 289-290, 1977.

182. Conway J. A vascular abnormality in hypertension. Circulation 27: 520-529, 1963.

183. Conway J. Changes in sodium balance and hemodynamics during development of experimental renal hypertension in dogs. Circ Res 22: 763-767, 1968.

184. Conway J , Hatton R. Development of deoxycorticosterone acetate hypertension in the dog. Circ Res 43(Suppl I): 82-86, 1978.

185. Conway J, Hatton R, Keddie J. Effect of converting enzyme inhibitor and saralasin on the reflex control of blood pressure. Clin Sci Molec Med 54: 5P-6P, 1978.

186. Conway J, Hatton R, Keddie J, Dawes P. The role of angiotensin in the control of blood pressure during sodium depletion. Hypertension 1: 402-409, 1979.

187. Conway J, Lauwers P. Haemodynamic and hypotensive effects of long-term therapy with chlorothiazide. Circulation 21: 21-27, 1960.

188. Cooper R, Soltero I, Liu K, Berkson D, Levinson S, Stamler J. The association between urinary sodium excretion and blood pressure in children. Circulation 62: 97-104, 1980.

189. Cowley AW Jr, DeClue JW. Quantification of baroreceptor influence on arterial pressure changes seen in primary angiotensin-induced hypertension in dogs. Circ Res 39: 779-787, 1976.

190. Cowley AW Jr, Guyton AC. Quantification of intermediate steps in the renin-angiotensin-vasoconstrictor feedback loop in the dog. Circ Res 30: 557-566, 1972.

191. Cowley AW Jr, Guyton AC. Baroreceptor reflex effects on transient and steady-state hemodynamics of salt-loading hypertension in dogs. Circ Res 36: 536-546, 1975.

192. Cowley AW Jr, Liard JF, Guyton AC. Role of the

baroreceptor reflex in daily control of arterial blood pressure and other variables in dogs. Circ Res 32: 564-576, 1973.

193. Cowley AW Jr, Lohmeier TE. Changes in renal vascular sensitivity and arterial pressure associated with sodium intake during long-term intrarenal norepinephrine infusion in dogs. Hypertension 1: 549-558, 1979.

194. Cowley AW Jr, McCaa RE. Acute and chronic dose-response relationships for angiotensin, aldosterone and arterial pressure at varying levels of sodium intake. Circ Res 39: 788-797, 1976.

195. Cowley AW Jr, Switzer SJ, Guinn MM. Evidence and quantification of the vasopressin arterial pressure control system in the dog. Circ Res 46: 58-67, 1980.

196. Crafoord C, Nylin G. Congenital coarctation of the aorta and its surgical treatment. J Thorac Surg 14: 347-361, 1945.

197. Crane MG, Harris JJ, Johns VJ Jr. Hyporeninemic hypertension. Amer J Med 52: 457-466, 1972.

198. Crofton JT, Share L, Horovitz ZP. The effect of SQ 14225 on systolic blood pressure and urinary excretion of vasopressin in the developing spontaneously hypertensive rat. Hypertension 1: 462-467, 1979.

199. Crofton JT, Share L, Shade RE, Allen C, Tarnowski D. Vasopressin in the rat with spontaneous hypertension. Amer J Physiol 235: H361- H366, 1978.

200. Crofton JT, Share L, Shade RE, Lee-Kwon WJ, Manning M, Sawyer WH. The importance of vasopressin in the development and maintenance of DOC-salt hypertension in the rat. Hypertension 1: 31-38, 1979.

201. Dahl LK. Salt intake and hypertension. Diet Curr 2: 1-4, 1975.

202. Dahl LK, Heine M. Primary role of renal homographs in setting chronic blood pressure level in rats. Circ Res 36: 692-696, 1975.

203. Dahl LK, Heine M, Tassinari L. Role of genetic factors in susceptibility to experimental hypertension due to chronic excess salt ingestion. Nature 194: 480-482, 1962.

204. Dahl LK, Heine M, Tassinari L. Effects of chronic excess salt ingestion. Role of genetic factors in both DOCA-salt and renal hypertension. J Exp Med 118: 605-617, 1963.

205. Dahl LK, Heine M, Thompson K. Genetic influences of the kidneys on blood pressure. Circ Res 34: 94-101, 1974.

206. Dahl LK, Knudsen KD, Heine MA, Leitl GJ. Effects of chronic excess salt ingestion: Modification of experimental hypertension in the rat by variations in the diet. Circ Res 22: 11-18, 1968.

207. Dahl LK, Leitl G, Heine M. Influence of dietary potassium and sodium/potassium molar ratios on the development of salt hypertension. J Exp Med 136: 318-330, 1972.

208. Dahl LK, Silver L, Christie R. Role of salt in the fall of blood pressure accompanying reduction in obesity. New Eng J Med 258: 1186-1192, 1958.

209. Dargie HJ, Franklin SS, Reid JL. Central and peripheral noradrenaline in the kidney model of renovascular hypertension in the rat. Brit J Pharmacol 61: 213-215, 1977.

210. Dargie HJ, Franklin SS, Reid JL. Plasma noradrenaline concentrations in experimental renovascular hypertension in the rat. Clin Sci Molec Med 52: 477-483, 1977.

211. Darke AC, Melnyk J, Nair PG, Gaskell P. Experimental aldosterone hypertension in the rat. Canad J Physiol Pharmacol 55: 681-690, 1977.

212. Davies DF, Shock NW. Age changes in glomerular filtration rate, effective renal plasma flow, and tubular excretory capacity in adult males. J Clin Invest 29: 496-507, 1950.

213. Davies MH. Is high pressure a psychosomatic disorder? J Chronic Dis 24: 239-258, 1971.

214. Davis JO, Freeman RH, Johnson JA, Spielman WS. Agents which block the action of the renin-angiotensin system. Circ Res 34: 279-285, 1974.

215. de Champlain J, Farley L, Cousineau D, van Ameringen M. Circulating catecholamine levels in human and experimental hypertension. Circ Res 38: 109-114, 1976.

216. de Champlain J, Krakoff LR, Axelrod J. Relationship between sodium intake and norepinephrine storage during the development of experimental hypertension. Circ Res 23: 479-491, 1968.

217. de Champlain J, van Amerigen MR. Regulation of blood pressure by sympathetic nerve fibers and adrenal medulla in normotensive and hypertensive rats. Circ Res 31: 617-628, 1972.

218. de Swiet M, Dickinson CJ. The delayed pressor response to small doses of intravenous noradrenaline in conscious rabbits. J Physiol 205: 515-526, 1969.

219. DeClue JW, Guyton AC, Cowley AW Jr, Coleman TG, Norman RA Jr, McCaa RE. Subpressor angiotensin infusion, renal sodium handling, and salt-induced hypertension in the dog. Circ Res 43: 503-512, 1978.

220. DeForrest JM, Davis JO, Freeman RH, Watkins BE, Stephens GA. Separate renal function studies in conscious dogs with renovascular hypertension. Amer J Physiol 235: F310-F316, 1978.

221. deJong W, Lovenberg W, Sjoerdsma A. Increased plasma renin activity in the spontaneously hypertensive rat. Proc Soc Exp Med Biol 139: 1213-1216, 1972.

222. del Greco F, Shere J, Simon NM. Hemodynamic effects of hemodialysis in chronic renal failure. Trans Amer Soc Art Intern Org 10: 353-355, 1964.

223. DeQuattro V, Miura Y, Lurvey A, Cosgrove M, Mendez R. Increase plasma catecholamine concentration and vas deferens norepinephrine biosynthesis in men with elevated blood pressure. Circ Res 36: 118-126, 1975.

224. deWardener HE, Mills IH, Clapham WF, Hayter CJ. Studies on the efferent mechanism of the sodium diuresis which follows the administration of intravenous saline in the dog. Clin Sci 21: 249-258, 1961.

225. DiBona GF. Neurogenic regulation of renal tubular sodium reabsorption. Amer J Physiol 233: F73-F81, 1977.

226. DiBona GF, Rios LL. Mechanism of exaggerated diuresis in spontaneously hypertensive rats. Amer J Physiol 235: F409-F416, 1978.

227. Dickinson CJ, de Swiet M. Slowly developing pressor response to small amounts of noradrenaline in rabbits. Lancet 1: 986-987, 1967.

228. Dickinson CJ, Lawrence JR. A slowly developing pressor response to small concentrations of angiotensin. Its bearing on pathogenesis of chronic renal hypertension. Lancet 1: 1354-1356, 1963.

229. Dickinson CJ, Shepard P. A digital computer model of the systemic circulation and kidney, for studying renal and circulatory interactions involving electrolytes and body fluid compartments ('MacPee'). J Physiol 216: 11-12, 1971.

230. Dickinson CJ, Yu R. Mechanisms involved in the progressive pressor response to very small amounts of angiotensin in conscious rabbits. Circ Res 21(Suppl II): 157-163, 1967.

231. Dietz R, Haebara H, Luth B, Mast GJ, Schomig A, Gross F. Antihypertensive measures and their consequences in malignant hypertensive rats. pp 3-19 in _Systematic Effects of Antihypertensive Agents_, ed MP _Sambhi_. Symposia Specialists, Miami, 1976.

232. Dietz R, Mast GJ, Haebare H, Schomig A, Luth JB, Gross F. The kidney after removal of one renal artery stenosis in the rat. Contrib Nephrol 3: 127-133, 1976.

233. Dietz R, Mast GJ, Mohring J, Vecsei P, Gless KH, Oster P, Gross F. Aldosterone and corticosterone production in renal hypertensive rats. Acta Endocrinol 79: 317-328, 1975.

234. Dietz R, Schomig A, Haebara H, Mann JFE, Rascher W, Luth JB, Grunherz N, Gross F. Studies on the pathogenesis of spontaneous hypertension of rats. Circ Res 43(Suppl I): 98-106, 1978.

235. Dlouha H, Krecek J, Zicha J. Hypertension in rats with hereditary diabetes insipidus. Pflueger Arch 369: 177-182, 1977.

236. Doba N, Reis DJ. Acute fulminating neurogenic hypertension produced by brainstem lesions in rat. Circ Res 32: 584-593, 1973.

237. Doba N, Reis DJ. Role of central and perophei al adrenergic mechanisms in neurogenic hypertension produced by brainstem lesions in the rat. Circ Res 34: 293-301, 1974.

238. Dole VP, Dahl LK, Cotzias GC, Eder HA, Krebs ME. Dietary treatment of hypertension. Clinical and metabolic studies of patients on the rice diet. J Clin Invest 29: 1189-1206, 1950.

239. Dollery CT, Miyamori I. Indomethacin and the hypotensive action of captopril in DOCA salt hypertensive rats. Brit J Pharmacol 68: P117-P118, 1980.

240. Dominguez R. Effect on the blood pressure of the rabbit of arteriosclerosis and nephritis caused by uranium. Arch Path 5: 577-606, 1928.

241. Dorr LD, Brody MJ. Preliminary observations on the role of the sympathetic nervous system in the development and maintenance of experimental renal hypertension. Proc Soc Exp Biol Med 123: 155-158, 1966.

242. Douglas BH, Guyton AC, Langston JB, Bishop VS. Hypertension caused by salt loading : II. Fluid volume and tissue pressure changes. Amer J Physiol 207: 669-671, 1964.

243. Douglas BH, Langford HG, McCaa RE. Response of mineralocorticoid hypertensive animals to an angiotensin I converting enzyme inhibitor. Proc Soc Exp Biol Med 161: 86-87, 1979.

244. Doyle AE, Duffy SG. Sodium balance and plasma renin

activity during the development of the two-kidney Goldblatt hypertension in rats. Clin Exp Pharmacol Physiol 7: 293-304, 1980.

245. Doyle AE, Jerums G, Johnson CI, Louis WJ. Plasma renin levels and vascular complications in hypertension. Brit Med J 2: 206-207, 1973.

246. Du Vigneaud V, Gish DT, Katsoyannis PG, Hess GP. Synthesis of pressor-antidiuretic hormone, arginine-vasopressin. J Amer Chem Soc 80: 3355-3358, 1958.

247. Du Vigneaud V, Lawler HC, Popenoe EA. Enzymatic cleavage of glycinamide from vasopressin and a proposed structure for this pressor-antidiuretic hormone of the posterior pituitary. J Amer Chem Soc 75: 4880-4881, 1953.

248. Dunn MJ, Tannen RL. Low renin essential hypertension. pp 349-364 in Hypertension: Physiopathology and Treatment, eds J Genest, E Koiw, O Kuchel. McGraw-Hill, New York, 1977.

249. Dustan HP, Poutasse EF, Corcoran AC, Page IH. Separated renal functions in patients with renal artery disease, pyelonephritis, and essential hypertension. Circulation 23: 34-41, 1961.

250. Dustan HR, Tarazi RC, Bravo EL. Diuretic and diet treatment of hypertension. Arch Intern Med 133: 1007-1013, 1974.

251. Dustan HP, Tarazi RC, Bravo EL, Dart RA. Plasma and extracellular fluid volumes in hypertension. Circ Res 32(Suppl I): 73-81, 1973.

252. Dyer AR. An analysis of the relationship of systolic blood pressure, serum cholesterol, and smoking to 14-year mortality in the Chicago peoples gas company study. J Chron Dis 28: 565-670, 1975.

253. Eckberg DL. Carotid baroreflex function in young men with borderline blood pressure elevation. Circulation 59: 632-636, 1979.

254. Eich Rh, Peters RJ, Cuddy RP, Smulyan H, Lyons RH. The hemodynamics in labile hypertension. Amer Heart J 63: 188-195, 1962.

255. Ekas RD Jr, Lokhandwala MF. Sympathetic nerve function and vascular reactivity in DOCA-salt hypertensive rats. Amer J Physiol 239: R303-R308, 1980.

256. Elliot DF, Peart WS. Amino acid sequence in a hypertensin. Nature 177: 527-528, 1956.

257. Ellis CN, Julius S. Role of central blood volume in hyperkinetic borderline hypertension. Brit Heart J 35: 450-455, 1973.

258. Engelman K, Portnoy B, Lovenberg W. A sensitive and specific double isotope derivative method for determination of catecholamines in biological specimens. Amer J Med Sci 255: 259-268, 1968.

259. Engelman K, Portnoy B, Sjoerdsma A. Plasma catecholamine concentrations in patients with hypertension. Circ Res 27(Suppl I): 141-145, 1970.

260. Erinoff L, Heller A, Oparil S. Prevention of hypertension in the SH rat: effect of differential central catecholamine depletion. Pro Soc Exp Med 150: 748-754, 1975.

261. Ernst CB, Daugherty ME, Kotchen TA. Relationship between collateral development and renin in experimental renal arterial stenosis. Surgery 80: 252-258, 1976.

262. Esler MD, Julius S, Randall OS, Ellis CN, Kashima T. Relation of renin status to neurogenic vascular resistance in borderline hypertension. Amer J Cardiol 36: 708-715, 1975.

263. Esler MD, Julius S, Zweifler A, Randall O, Harburg E, Gardiner H, DeQuattro V. Mild high-renin essential hypertension: neurogenic human hypertension? New Eng J Med 296: 405-411, 1977.

264. Esler MD, Nestel PJ. Essential hypertension with symptoms of hyperkinetic circulation. Med J Aust 2: 253-257, 1973.

265. Esler MD, Nestel PJ. Renin and sympathetic nervous system responsiveness to adrenergic stumuli in essential hypertension. Amer J Cardiol 32: 643-649, 1973.

266. Falch DK, Odegaard AE, Norman N. Decreased renal plasma flow during propranolol treatment in essential hypertension. Acta Med Scand 205: 91-95, 1979.

267. Falkner B, Onesti G, Angelakos ET, Fernandes M, Langman C. Cardiovascular response to mental stress in normal adolescents with hypertensive parents. Hypertension 1: 23-30, 1979.

268. Falls F, Armanini D, Maragno I, Mantero F. Plasma renin activity in coarctation of the aorta before and after surgical correction. Brit Heart J 40: 1415-1418, 1978.

269. Fan JSK, Coghlan JP, Denton DA, Scoggins BA, Whitworth JA. Blood pressure and metabolic effects of ACTH in anephric sheep. Clin Exp Pharmacol Physiol 5: 673-677, 1978.

270. Farris EJ, Yeakel EH, Medoff HS. Development of hypertension in emotional gray Norway rats after air blasting. Amer J Physiol 144: 331-333, 1945.

271. Feinleib M, Garrison R, Borhani N, Rosenman R, Christian J. Studies of hypertension in twins. pp 3-17 in Epidemiology and Control of Hypertension, ed O Paul, Stratten Intercontinential Medical Book Corp, New York, 1975.

272. Fekete A. Permanent hypertension induced by ligation of one renal artery in the dog. Acta Acad Sci Hung 27: 191-204, 1970.

273. Feldschuh J, Enson Y. Prediction of the normal blood volume: Relation of blood volume to body habitus. Circulation 56: 605-612, 1977.

274. Ferlinz J. Right ventricular performance in essential hypertension. Circulation 61: 156-162, 1980.

275. Ferrario CM. Contribution of cardiac output and peripheral resistance to experimental renal hypertension. Amer J Physiol 226: 711-717, 1974.

276. Ferrario CM, Dickinson CJ, McCubbin JW. Central vasomotor stimulation by angiotensin. Clin Sci 39: 239-245, 1970.

277. Ferrario CM, Gildenberg PL, McCubbin JW. Cardiovascular effects of angiotensin mediated by the central nervous system. Circ Res 30: 257-262, 1972.

278. Ferrario CM, McCubbin JW. Renal blood flow and perfusion pressure before and after development of renal hypertension. Amer J Physiol 224: 102-109, 1973.

279. Ferrario CM, McCubbin JW, Page IH. Hemodynamic characteristics of chronic experimental neurogenic hypertension in unanesthesized dog. Circ Res 24: 911-922, 1969.

280. Ferrario CM, Page IH, McCubbin JW. Increased cardiac output as a contributory factor in experimental renal hypertension in dogs. Circ Res 27: 799-810, 1970.

281. Ferreira SH. A bradykinin-potentiating factor present in the venom of the Bothrops jararaca. Brit J Pharmacol 24: 163-169, 1965.

282. Ferreira SH, Bartelt DC, Greene LJ. Isolation of bradykinin-potentiating peptides from Bothrops jararaca venom. Biochemistry 9: 2583-2593, 1970.

283. Ferreira SH, Greene LJ, Alabaster VA, Bakhle YS, Vane JR. Activity of various fractions of bradykinin potentiating factor against angiotensin I converting enzyme. Nature 255: 379-380, 1970.

284. Ferreira SH, Vane JR. The disappearance of bradykinin and eledoisin in the circulation and vascular beds of the cat. Brit J Pharmacol Chemother 30: 417-424, 1967.

285. Ferrone RA, Antonaccio MJ. Prevention of the development of spontaneous hypertension in rats by captopril (SQ 14225). Eur J Pharmacol 60: 131-137, 1979.

286. Finch L. Cardiovascular reactivity in the experimental hypertensive rat. Brit J Pharmacol 42: 56-65, 1971.

287. Finch L. An increased reactivity in hypertensive rats unaffected by prolonged antihypertensive therapy. Brit J Pharmacol 54: 437-443, 1975.

288. Finch L, Cohen M, Horst WD. Effects of 6-hydroxydopamine at birth on the development of hypertension in the rat. Life Sci 13: 1403-1410, 1973.

289. Finch L, Leach GDH. Does the adrenal medulla contribute to the maintenance of experimental hypertension. Europ J Pharmacol 11: 388-391, 1970.

290. Fink GD, Brody MJ. Renal vascular resistance and reactivity in the spontaneously hypertensive rat. Amer J Physiol 237: F128-F132, 1979.

291. Fink GD, Buggy J, Johnson AK, Brody MJ. Prevention of steroid-salt hypertension in the rat by anterior forebrain lesions. Circulation 56(Suppl II): 242, 1977.

292. Fink GD, Kennedy F, Bryan WJ, Werber A. Pathogenesis of hypertension in rats with chronic aortic baroreceptor deafferentation. Hypertension 2: 319-325, 1980.

293. Fink GD, Takeshita A, Mark AL, Brody MJ. Determinants of renal vascular resistance in the Dahl strain of genetically hypertensive rat. Hypertension 2: 274-280, 1980.

294. Finnerty FA Jr. Relationship of extracellular fluid volume to the development of drug resistance in the hypertensive patient. Amer Heart J 81: 563-565, 1971.

295. Fisher ER, Klein HZ. Effect of renal hypertension in sodium deficient rats on juxtaglomerular index and zona glomerulosa. Proc Soc Exp Biol Med 113: 37-39, 1963.

296. Fisher ER, Pirog J. Renal arteriolar obstruction without hypertension. Nephron 16: 433-438, 1976.

297. Fitzsimons JT. Angiotensin, thirst, and sodium appetite: retrospect and prospect. Fed Proc 37: 2669-2675, 1978.

298. Fletcher A. The effect of weight reduction upon the blood pressure of obese hypertensive women. Quart J Med 91: 331-345, 1954.

299. Fletcher PJ, Angus JA, Oliver JR, Korner PI. Effects of the angiotensin antagonist P-113 in chronic renal hypertension. Clin Exp Pharmacol Physiol 2: 428-429, 1975.

300. Fletcher PJ, Korner PI, Angus JA, Oliver JR. Changes in cardiac output and total peripheral resistance during the development if renal hypertension in the rabbit. 39: 633-639, 1976.

301. Floyer MA. The effects of nephrectomy and adrenalectomy upon the blood pressure in hypertensive and normotensive rats. Clin Sci 10: 405-421, 1951.

302. Floyer MA. Further studies on the mechanism of experimental hypertension in the rat. Clin Sci 14: 163-181, 1955.

303. Folkow B. The hemodynamic consequences of adaptive structural changes of the resistance vessels in hypertension. Clin Sci 41: 1-12, 1971.

304. Folkow B. Role of the vascular factor in hypertension. Contr Nephol 8: 81-94, 1977.

305. Folkow B, Grimby G, Thulesius O. Adoptive structural changes of the vascular walls in hypertension and their relation to the control of the peripheral resistance. Acta Physiol Scand 44: 255-272, 1958.

306. Folkow B, Gurevich M, Hallback M, Lundgren Y, Weiss L. The hemodynamic consequences of regional hypotension in spontaneously hypertensive and normotensive rats. Acta Physiol Scand 83: 532-541, 1971.

307. Folkow B, Hallback M, Lundgren Y, Weiss L. The effects of "immunosympathectomy" on blood pressure and vascular reactivity in normal and spontaneously hypertensive rats. Acta Physiol Scand 84: 512-523, 1972.

308. Folkow B. Gothberg G, Lundin S, Ricksten SE. Structural 'resetting' of the renal vascular bed in spontaneously hypertensive rats. Acta Physiol Scand 100: 270-272, 1977.

309. Folkow BUG, Hallback MIL. Physiopathology of spontaneous hypertension in rats. pp 507-529 in

Hypertension. Physiopathology and Treatment, eds J Genest, E Koiw, O Kuchel. McGraw-Hill, New York, 1977.

310. Fouad FM, Ceimo JMK, Tarazi RC, Bravo EL. Contrasts and similarities of acute hemodynamic responses to specific antagonism of angiotensin II ((Sar-1, Thr-8) A II) and to inhibition of converting enzyme (captopril). Circulation 61: 163-169, 1980.

311. Fourcade JC, Navar LG, Guyton AC. Possibility that angiotensin resulting from unilateral kidney disease affects contralateral renal function. Nephron 8: 1-16, 1971.

312. Freed MD, Rocchini A, Rosenthal A, Nadas AS, Castaneda AR. Exercise-induced hypertension after surgical repair of coarctation of the aorta. Amer J Cardiol 43: 253-258, 1979.

313. Freeman NE, Page H. Hypertension produced by constriction of the renal artery in sympathectomized dogs. Amer Heart J 14: 405-414 1937.

314. Freeman RH, Davis JO, Fullerton D. Chronic ACTH administration and the development of hypertension in rats. Proc Soc Exp Biol Med 163: 473-477, 1980.

315. Freeman RH, Davis JO, Varsano-Aharon N, Ulick S, Weinberger MH. Control of aldosterone secretion in the spontaneously hypertensive rat. Circ Res 37: 66-71, 1975.

316. Freeman RH, Davis JO, Watkins BE. Development of chronic perinephritic hypertension in dogs without volume expansion. Amer J Physiol 233: F278-F281, 1977.

317. Freeman RH, Davis JO, Watkins BE, Stephens GA, DeForrest JM. Effects of continuous converting enzyme blockade on renovascular hypertension in the rat. Amer J Physiol 236: F21-F24, 1979.

318. Freis ED. Hemodynamics of hypertension. Physiol Rev 40: 27-54, 1960.

319. Freis ED, Wilson IM. Potentiating effect of chlorothiazide (diuril) in combination with antihypertensive agents. Med Ann DC 26: 468 and

516, 1957.

320. Friedman M, Selzer A, Rosenblum H. The renal blood flow in hypertension. JAMA 117, 92-95, 1941.

321. Friedman R, Dahl LK. The effect of chronic conflict on the blood pressure of rats with a genetic susceptability to experimental hypertension. Psychosomatic Med 37: 402-416, 1975.

322. Friedman R, Iwai J. Genetic predisposition and stress-induced hypertension. Science 193: 161-162, 1976.

323. Friedman R, Iwai J. Dietary sodium, psychic stress, and genetic predisposition to experimental hypertension. Proc Soc Exp Biol Med 155: 449-452, 1977.

324. Friedman R, Tassinari LM, Heine M, Iwai J. Differential development of salt-induced and renal hypertension in Dahl hypertension-sensitive rats after neonatal sympathectomy. Clin Exp Hyperten 1: 779-799, 1979.

325. Friedman SM, Friedman CL. Salt and water distribution in hereditary and in induced hypothalamic diabetes insipidus in the rats. Canad J Physiol Pharmacol 43: 699-705, 1965.

326. Friedman SM, Friedman CL. Cell permeability, sodium transport, and the hypertensive process in the rat. Circ Res 39: 433-441, 1976.

327. Friedman SM, Polley JR, Friedman CL. The effect of deoxycorticosterone acetate on blood pressure, renal function, and electrolyte pattern in the intact rat. J Exp Med 87: 329-338, 1948.

328. Frohlich ED, Dustan HP, Page IH. Hyperdynamic beta-adrenergic circulatory state. Arch Intern Med 117: 614-619, 1966.

329. Frohlich ED, Tarazi RC, Dustan HP, Page IH. The paradox of beta-adrenergic blockade in hypertension. Circulation 37: 417-423, 1968.

330. Frohlich ED, Ulrych M, Tarazi RC, Dustan HP, Page IH. A hemodynamic comparison of essential and

renovascular hypertension. Circulation 35: 289-297, 1967.

331. Fukiyama K, McCubbin JW, Page IH. Chronic hypertension elicited by infusion of angiotensin into vertebral arteries of unanesthetized dogs. Clin Sci 40: 283-291, 1971.

332. Fukuda M, Green JA Jr, Vander AJ. Plasma renin activity during development of experimental antiserium glomerular nephritis. J Lab Clin Med 71: 148-152, 1968.

333. Funder JW, Blair-West JR, Cain MC, Catt KJ, Coghlan JP, Denton DA, Nelson JF, Scoggins BA, Wright RD. Circulatory and humoral changes in the reversal of renovascular hypertension in sheep by unclipping the renal artery. Circ Res 27: 249-258, 1970.

334. Fyhrquist F, Kala R, Standerskiold-Nordenstan CG, Eisalo A. Angiotensin II plasma levels in hypertensive patients. Acta Med Scand 192: 507-511, 1972.

335. Galosy RA, Gaebelein CJ. Cardiovascular adaptation to environmental stress: Its role in the development of hypertension, responsible mechanisms, and hypothesis. Biobehav Rev 1: 165-175, 1977.

336. Ganguli M, Tobian L, Dahl L. Low renal papillary plasma flow in both Dahl and Kyoto rats with spontaneous hypertension. Circ Res 39: 337-341, 1976.

337. Ganguli M, Tobian L, Iwai J. Cardiac output and peripheral resistance in strains of rats sensitive and resistant to NaCl hypertension. Hypertension 1: 3-7, 1979.

338. Garay RP, Dagher G, Pernollet MG, Devynck MA, Meyer P. Inherited defect in a Na+, K+-co-transport system in erythrocytes from essential hypertensive patients. Nature 284: 281-283, 1980.

339. Garay RP, Elghozi JL, Dagher G, Meyer P. Laboratory distinction between essential and secondary hypertension by measurement of erythrocyte cation fluxes. New Eng J Med 302: 769-771, 1980.

340. Garner D, Laks MM. The hemodynamic effects of long-term subhypertensive infusion of norepinephrine in the conscious dog. Physiologist 18: 224, 1975.

341. Gavras H, Brunner HR, Laragh JH, Vaughan ED Jr, Koss M, Cote LJ, Gavras I. Malignant hypertension resulting from deoxycorticosterone acetate and salt excess. Circ Res 36: 300-309, 1975.

342. Gavras H, Brunner HR, Thurston H, Laragh JH. Reciprocation of renin dependency with sodium volume dependency in renal hypertension. Science 188: 1316-1317, 1975.

343. Gavras H, Brunner HR, Turini GA, Kershaw GR, Tifft CP, Cuttelod S, Gavras I, Vukovich RA, McKinstry DN. Antihypertensive effect of the oral angiotensin converting-enzyme inhibitor (SQ 14225) in man. New Eng J Med 298: 991-995, 1978.

344. Gavras H, Brunner HR, Vaughan ED Jr, Laragh JH. Angiotensin-sodium interaction in blood pressure maintenance of renal hypertensive and normotensive rats. Science 180: 1369-1372, 1973.

345. Gavras H, Liang CS. Acute renovascular hypertension in conscious dogs. Interaction of the renin-angiotension system and sympathetic nervous system in systemic hemodynamics and regional blood flow responses. Circ Res 47: 356-365, 1980.

346. Geddes LA. <u>The Direct and Indirect Measurement of Blood Pressure</u>. Year Book Medical Publishers, Chicago, 1970.

347. Giachetti A, Rubinstein R, Clark TL. Noradrenaline storage in deoxycorticosterone-saline hypertensive rats. Europ J Pharmacol 57: 99-106, 1979.

348. Gilmore JP. Pentobarbital sodium anesthesia in the dog. Amer J Physiol 209: 404-408, 1965.

349. Giovannetti S, Bigalli A, Balestri PL. On the pathogenesis of the renoprival hypertension in dogs. Experientia 21: 288-289, 1965.

350. Goldblatt H, Gross J, Hanzel RF. Studies on experimental hypertension. II. The effect of resection of splanchnic nerves on experimental renal

hypertension. J Exp Med 65: 233-241, 1937.

351. Goldblatt H, Kahn JR, Bayless F, Simon MA. Studies on experimental hypertension. XI. The effect of excision of the carotid sinuses on experimental hypertension produced by renal ischemia. J Exp Med 71: 175-185, 1940.

352. Goldblatt H, Kahn JR, Hanzal RF. Studies on experimental hypertension. IX. The effect on blood pressure of constriction of the abdominal aorta above and below the site of origin of both main renal arteries. J Exp Med 69: 649-674, 1939.

353. Goldblatt H, Lynch J, Hanzal RF, Summerville WW. Studies on experimental hypertension. I. The production of persistent elevation of systolic blood pressure by means of renal ischemia. J Exp Med 59: 347-379, 1934.

354. Goldring W, Chasis H, Ranges HA, Smith HW. Effective renal blood flow in subjects with essential hypertension. J Clin Invest 20: 637-653, 1941.

355. Gomez AH, Hoobler SW, Blaquier P. Effect of addition and removal of a kidney transplant in renal and adrenocortical hypertensive rats. Circ Res 8: 464-472, 1960.

356. Gomez DM. Evaluation of renal resistances, with special reference to changes in hypertension. J Clin Invest 30: 1143-1155, 1951.

357. Gonick HC, Coburn JW, Rubini ME, Maxwell MH, Kleeman CR. Studies of experimental renal failure in dogs. II. Effect of 5/6 nephrectomy on sodium conserving ability of residual nephrons. J Lab Clin Med 64: 269-276, 1964.

358. Gordon FJ, Brody MJ, Fink GD, Buggy J, Johnson AK. Role of central catecholamines in the control of blood pressure and drinking behavior. Brain Res 178: 161-173, 1979.

359. Gordon FJ, Haywood JR, Johnson AK, Brody MJ. Effect of anteroventral third ventricle (AV3V) lesions on the development of hypertension in spontaneously hypertensive rats. Fed Proc 38: 1233, 1979.

360. Gordon RD, Mortimer RH, Saar N. Failure of methyclothiazide to lower home blood pressure level in "essential" hypertensive and normotensive young men, despite significant plasma volume contraction. Europ J Clin Pharmacol 12: 403-408, 1977.

361. Gordon T, Kannel WB. Predisposition to atherosclerosis in the head, heart and legs: The Framingham Study. JAMA 221: 661-666, 1972.

362. Goss JE, Alfrey AC, Vogel JHK, Holmes JH. Hemodynamic changes during hemodialysis. Trans Amer Soc Art Intern Org 13: 68-74, 1967.

363. Goss LZ, Rosa R, O'Brien WM, Ayers CR, Wood JE. Predicting death from renal failure in primary hypertension. Arch Intern Med 124: 160-164, 1969.

364. Gothberg G, Lundin S, Ricksten SE, Folkow B. Apparent and true vascular resistance to flow in SHR and NCR kidneys as related to the pre/postglomerular resistance ratio. Acta Physiol Scand 105: 282-294, 1979.

365. Green DM, Johanson AD, Bridges WC, Lehmann AH. Stages of salt excretion in essential hypertension. Circulation 9: 416-424, 1954.

366. Greenberg S, Bohr DF. Venous smooth muscle in hypertension: Enhanced contractility of portal veins from spontaneously hypertensive rats. Circ Res 36(Suppl I): 208-215, 1975.

367. Greene RW, Sapirstein LA. Total body sodium, potassium, and nitrogen in rats made hypertensive by subtotal nephrectomy. Amer J Physiol 169: 343-349, 1952.

368. Gresson CR. Suppressed renin levels in the genetically hypertensive rat. Proc Univ Otago Med Sch 50: 51-52, 1972.

369. Gresson CR, Bird DL, Simpson FO. Plasma volume, extracellular fluid volume and exchangeable sodium concentrations in the New Zealand strain of genetically hypertensive rat. Clin Sci 44: 349-358, 1973.

370. Gresson CR, Bird DL, Simpson FO. Plasma volume,

total body sodium and total body water volume in young genetically hypertensive rats. Life Sci 12: 393-399, 1973.

371. Gribbin B, Pickering TG, Sleight P, Peto R. Effect of age and high blood pressure on baroreflex sensitivity in man. Circ Res 29: 424-431, 1971.

372. Grim CE, Luft FC, Fineberg NS, Weinberger MH. Responses to volume expansion and contraction in categorized hypertensive and normotensive man. Hypertension 1: 476-485, 1979.

373. Grim CE, Luft FC, Miller JZ, Brown PL, Gannon MA, Weinberger MH. Effects of sodium loading and depletion in normotensive first-degree relatives of essential hypertensives. J Lab Clin Med 94: 764-771, 1979.

374. Grim CE, Miller JZ, Luft FC, Christian JC, Weinberger MH. Genetic influences on renin, aldosterone, and the renal excretion of sodium and potassium following volume expansion and contraction in normal man. Hypertension 1: 583-590, 1979.

375. Grobecker H, Roizen MF, Weise V, Saavedra JM, Kopin IJ. Sympathoadrenal medullary activity in young, spontaneously hypertensive rats. Nature 258: 267, 1975.

376. Grodins FS. Integrated cardiovascular physiology: A mathematical synthesis of cardiac output and blood vessel hemodynamics. Quant Rev Biol 34: 93-116, 1959.

377. Grollman A. Physiological variations in the cardiac output in man. IV. The effect of psychic disturbances on the cardiac output, pulse, blood pressure, and oxygen consumption of man. Amer J Physiol 89: 584-588, 1929.

378. Grollman A. A simplified procedure for inducing chronic renal hypertension in the mammal. Proc Soc Exp Med Biol 57: 102-104, 1944.

379. Grollman A. Experimental hypertension in the dog. Amer J Physiol 147: 647-653, 1946.

380. Grollman A, Harrison TR, Williams JR Jr. The effect

of various sterol derivatives on the blood pressure of the rat. J Pharmacol Exp Ther 69: 149-155, 1940.

381. Grollman A, Shapiro AP. The volume of the extracellular fluid in experimental and human hypertension. J Clin Invest 32: 312-316, 1953.

382. Grollman A, Turner LB, Levitch M, Hill D. Hemodynamics of bilaterally nephrectomized dog subject to intermittent peritoneal lavage. Amer J Physiol 165: 167-172, 1951.

383. Gross F, Lazar J, Orth H. Inhibition of the renin-angiotensinogen reaction by pepstatin. Science 175: 656, 1972.

384. Gross F, Loustalot P, Meier R. Production of experimental hypertension by aldosterone. Acta Endocrinol 26: 417-423, 1957.

385. Gross RE. Surgical correction for coarctation of the aorta. Surgery 18: 673-678, 1945.

386. Guazzi M, Magrini F, Fiorentini C, Polese A. Role of the sympathetic nervous system in supporting cardiac function in essential arterial hypertension. Brit Heart J 35: 55-64, 1973.

387. Gupta TC, Wiggers CJ. Basic hemodynamic changes produced by aortic coarctation of different degrees. Circulation 3: 17-31, 1951.

388. Gutmann FD, Tagawa E, Haber E, Barger AC. Renal arterial pressure, renin secretion, and blood pressure control in trained dogs. Amer J Physiol 224: 66-72, 1973.

389. Guyton AC. Circulatory Physiology. III. Arterial Pressure and Hypertension. Saunders, Philadelphia, 1980.

390. Guyton AC, Batson HM, Smith CM, Armstrong GG. Method for studying competence of the body's blood pressure regulatory mechanisms and the effect of pressoreceptor denervation. Amer J Physiol 164: 360-368, 1951.

391. Guyton AC, Coleman TG. Long-term regulation of the circulation; Interrelationships with body fluid

volumes. pp 179-201 in Physical Bases of Circulatory Transport, Regulation and Exchange, eds EB Reeve, AC Guyton. Saunders, Philadelphia, 1967.

392. Guyton AC, Coleman TG. Quantitative analysis of the pathophysiology of hypertension. 24:(Suppl I): I1-I19, 1969.

393. Guyton AC, Coleman TG, Granger HJ. Circulation : Overall control. Ann Rev Physiol 34: 13-46, 1972.

394. Guyton AC, Jones CE, Coleman TG. Circulatory Physiology : Cardiac Output and its Regulation. Saunders, Philadelphia, 1973.

395. Haack D, Engel R, Vecsei P. The effect of chronic ACTH treatment on blood pressure and urinary excretion of steroids in the rat. Klin Woch 56(Suppl I): 183-186, 1978.

396. Haack D, Mohring J, Mohring B, Petri M, Hackenthal E. Comparative study on development of corticosterone and DOCA hypertension in rats. Amer J Physiol 233: F403-F411, 1977.

397. Haddy FJ, Overbeck HW. The role of humoral agents in volume expanded hypertension. Life Sci 19: 935-948, 1976.

398. Haddy FJ, Pamnani M, Clough D. Review. The sodium-potassium pump in volume expanded hypertension. Clin Exp Hyperten 1: 295-336, 1978.

399. Haeusler G, Finch L, Thoenen H. Central adrenergic neurons and the initiation and development of experimental hypertension. Experientia 28: 1200-1203, 1972.

400. Hall CE, Ayachi S, Hall O. Spontaneous hypertension in rats with hereditary hypothalamic diabetes insipidus (Brattleboro strain). Texas Rep Biol Med 31: 471-487, 1973.

401. Hall CE, Hall O. The comparative hypertensive activities of the acetates of D-aldosterone and deoxycorticosterone. Acta Endocrinol 54: 399-410, 1967.

402. Hall CE, Hall O. Interaction between

desoxycorticosterone treatment, fluid intake, sodium consumption, blood pressure, and organ changes in rats drinking water, saline, or sucrose solution. Canad J Physiol Pharmacol 47: 81-86, 1969.

403. Hall JE, Coleman TG, Guyton AC, Balfe JW, Salgado HC. Intrarenal role of angiotensin II and (des-Asp,1) angiotensin II. Amer J Physiol 236: F252-F259, 1979.

404. Hall JE, Guyton AC, Jackson TE, Coleman TG, Lohmeier TE, Trippodo NC. Control of glomerular filtration rate by renin-angiotensin system. Amer J Physiol 233: F366-F372, 1977.

405. Hall JE, Guyton AC, Salgado HC, McCaa RE, Balfe JW. Renal hemodynamics in acute and chronic angiotensin II hypertension. Amer J Physiol 235: F174-F179, 1978.

406. Hall JE, Guyton AC, Smith MJ Jr, Coleman TG. Blood pressure and renal function during chronic changes in sodium intake: role of angiotensin. Amer J Physiol 239: F271-F280, 1980.

407. Hall JE, Guyton AC, Smith MJ Jr, Coleman TG. Chronic blockade of angiotensin II formation during sodium deprivation. Amer J Physiol 237: F424-F432, 1979.

408. Hall JE, Morse CL, Smith MJ Jr, Young DB, Guyton AC. Control of arterial pressure and renal function during glucocorticoid excess in dogs. Hypertension 2: 139-148, 1980.

409. Hallback M, Gothberg G, Lundin S, Ricksten SE, Folkow B. Hemodynamic consequences of resistance vessel rarification and of changes in smooth muscle sensitivity. Acta Physiol Scand 97: 233-240, 1976.

410. Hallback M, Jones JV, Bianchi G, Folkow B. Cardiovascular control in the Milan strain of spontaneously hypertensive rat at "rest" and during acuate mental "stress". Acta Physiol Scand 99: 208-216, 1977.

411. Hallback-Nordlander M, Noresson E, Lundgren Y. Hemodynamic alterations after reversal of renal hypertension in rats. Clin Sci 57: 155-175, 1979.

412. Hallback-Nordlander M, Noresson E, Thoren P. Hemodynamic consequences of left ventricular hypertrophy in spontaneously hypertensive rats. Amer J Cardiol 44: 986-993, 1979.

413. Hallbook T, Lundstrom NR, Mortensson W. Peak blood flow in the calves of children with aortic coarctation. Pediatr Cardiol 1: 35-37, 1979.

414. Hamilton M, Pickering GW, Roberts JAF, Sowry GSC. The etiology of essential hypertension. 4. The role of inheritance. Clin Sci 13: 273-304, 1954.

415. Hansson L. Beta-adrenergic blockade in essential hypertension. Acta Med Scand Suppl 550: 1-30, 1973.

416. Harburg E, Erfurt JC, Hauenstein LS, Chape C, Schull WJ, Schork MA. Socio-ecological stress, suppressed hostility, skin color, and black-white male blood pressure: Detroit. Phychosom Med 35: 276-296, 1973.

417. Harris PJ, Young JA. Dose-dependent stimulation and inhibition of proximal tubular sodium reabsorption by angiotensin II in the rat kidney. Pflueger Arch 367: 295-297, 1977.

418. Harris RC, Ayers CR. Renal hemodynamics and plasma renin activity after renal artery constriction in conscious dogs. Circ Res 31: 520-530, 1972.

419. Hartman HR, Ghrist DG. Blood pressure and weight. Arch Intern Med 44: 877-881, 1929.

420. Hatzinikolaou P, Gavras H, Brunner HR, Gavras I. Sodium-induced elevation of blood pressure in the anephric state. Science 209: 935-936, 1980.

421. Havlik RJ, Garrison RJ, Feinleib M, Padgett S, Castelli WP, McNamara PM. Evidence for additional blood pressure correlates in adults 20-56 years old. Circulation 61: 710-715, 1980.

422. Havlik RJ, Garrison RJ, Katz SH, Ellison RC, Feinlieb M, Myrianthopoulos NC. Detection of genetic variance in blood pressure of seven-year-old twins. Amer J Epidem 109: 512-516, 1979.

423. Hayman JM Jr, Shumway NP, Dunke P, Miller M.

Experimental hyposthenuria. J Clin Invest 18: 195-212, 1939.

424. Hayes CG, Tyroler HA, Cassel JC. Family aggregation of blood pressure in Evans County, Georgia. Arch Intern Med 128: 965-975, 1971.

425. Hayslett JP, Kashgarian M, Epstein FH. Functional correlates of compensatory renal hypertrophy. J Clin Invest 47: 774-782, 1968.

426. Hayslett JP, Kashgarian M, Epstein FH. Mechanism of change in the excretion of sodium per nephron when renal mass is reduced. J Clin Invest 48: 1002-1006, 1969.

427. Heine BE, Sainsbury P, Chynoweth RC. Hypertension and emotional disturbance. J Psychiat Res 7: 119-130, 1969.

428. Hejl Z. Changes in cardiac output and peripheral resistance during simple stimuli influencing blood pressure. Cardiologia 31: 375-381, 1957.

429. Hejl Z, Hofman J, Ulrych M. Essential hypertension. Hemodynamic and renal response to hypertonic sodium-chloride infusion. Lancet 1: 515-516, 1962.

430. Helmchen V, Kneissler V, Churchill P, Peters-Haefeli L, Schaechtelin G, Peters G. Plasma renin activity in renal hypertensive rats. Pflueger Arch 332: 232-238, 1972.

431. Helmchen V, Kneissler V, Liard JF, Peters G. Renin secretion in the earliest stage of Goldblatt-type hypertension in rats. Klin Wschr 50: 841-844, 1972.

432. Hennekens CH, Jesse MJ, Klein BE, Gourley JE, Blumenthal S. Aggregation of blood pressure in infants and their siblings. Amer J Epidem 103: 457-463, 1976.

433. Henrich H, Hertel R, Assmann R. Structural differences in the mesentary microcirculation between normotensive and spontaneously hypertensive rats. Pfluegers Arch 375: 153-159, 1978.

434. Henry JP, Meehan JP, Stephens PM. The use of psychosocial stimuli to induce prolonged systolic

hypertension in mice. Psychosom Med 29: 408-432, 1967.

435. Henry JP, Stephens PM, Santisteban GA. A model of psychosocial hypertension showing reversibility and progression of cardiovascular complications. Circ Res 36: 156-164, 1975.

436. Herd JA, Morse WH, Kelleher RT, Jones LG. Arterial hypertension in the squirrel monkey during behavioral experiments. Amer J Physiol 217: 24-29, 1969.

437. Herlitz H, Lundin S, Ricksten SE, Gothberg G, Aurell M, Hallback M, Berglund G. Sodium balance and structural vascular changes in the kidney during development of hypertension in spontaneously hypertensive rats. Acta Med Scand S625: 111-115, 1979.

438. Hertel R, Henrich H. Microvascular pressures and permeability in spontaneously hypertensive and normotensive rats. Bibl Anat 18: 180-183, 1979.

439. Hertel R, Henrich H, Assmann R. Intravital measurement of arteriolar pressure and tangential wall stress in normotensive and spontaneously hypertensive rats (established hypertension). Experientia 34: 865-867, 1978.

440. Heymans C. Experimental arterial hypertension. New Eng J Med 219: 154-156, 1938.

441. Hickam JB, Cargill WH, Golden A. Cardiovascular reactions to emotional stimuli. Effect on the cardiac output, arteriovenous oxygen difference, arterial pressure, and peripheral resistance. J Clin Invest 27: 290-298, 1948.

442. Holland WW, Beresford SAA. Factors influencing blood pressure in children. pp 375-383 in _Epidemiology and Control in Hypertension_, ed O Paul, Stratten Intercontinental Medical Book Corp, New York, 1975.

443. Hollander W, Chobanian AV, Burrows BA. Body fluid and electrolyte composition in arterial hypertension. I. Studies in essential, renal and malignant hypertension. J Clin Invest 40: 408-415, 1961.

444. Hollander W, Kramsh DM, Farmelaut M, Madoff IM.

Arterial wall metabolism in experimental hypertension of coarctation of the aorta of short duration. J Clin Invest 47: 1221-1229, 1968.

445. Hollander W, Wilkins RW. Chlorothiazide : A new type of drug for the treatment of arterial hypertension. Boston Med Quart 8: 69-75, 1957.

446. Hollenberg NK, Adams DF. The renal circulation in hypertensive disease. Amer J Med 60: 773-784, 1976.

447. Hollenberg NK, Adams DF, Solomon H, Chenitz WR, Burges BM, Abrams HL, Merrill JP. Renal vascular tone in essential and secondary hypertension: hemodynamic and angiographic responses to vasodilators. Medicine 54: 29-44, 1975.

448. Hollenberg NK, Adams DF, Solomon HS, Rashid A, Abrams HL, Merrill JP. Senescence and the renal vasculature in normal man. Circ Res 34: 309-316, 1974.

449. Hollenberg NK, Borucki LJ, Adams DF. The renal vasculature in early essential hypertension: Evidence for a pathogenic role. Medicine 57: 167-178, 1978.

450. Hollenberg NK, Epstein M, Basch RI, Merrill JP. "No Man's Land" of the renal vasculature. Amer J Med 47: 845-854, 1969.

451. Hollenberg NK, Epstein M, Guttmann RD, Conroy M, Basch RI, Merrill JP. Effect of sodium balance on intrarenal distribution of blood flow in normal man. J Appl Physiol 28: 312-317, 1970.

452. Hollenberg NK, Solomon HS, Adams DF, Abrams HL, Merrill JP. Renal vascular responses to angiotensin and norepinephrine in normal man. Circ Res 31: 750-757, 1972.

453. Hollenberg NK, Swartz SL, Passan DR, Williams GH. Increased glomerular filtration rate after converting enzyme inhibition in essential hypertension. New Eng J Med 301: 9-12, 1979.

454. Hollenberg NK, Williams GH, Taub KJ, Ishikawa I, Brown C, Adams DF. Renal vascular response to interruption of the renin-angiotensin system in normal man. Kid Inter 12: 285-293, 1977.

455. Hollifield JW, Sherman K, Vander Zwagg R, Shand DG. Proposed mechanisms of propranolol's antihypertensive effect in essential hypertension. New Eng J Med 295: 68-73, 1976.

456. Honda K, Maekawa S, Tamura T, Uchiyama S, Suzuki K, Yashima O, Ozawa M, Takahashi E, Kimura T. The role of the peripheral sympathetic nerves and the adrenal medulla in maintaining blood pressure of essential hypertension. Jap Circ J 39: 591-595, 1975.

457. Hong Tai Eng FW, Huber-Smith M, McCann DS. The role of sympathetic activity in normal renin essential hypertension. Hypertension 2: 14-19, 1980.

458. Houck CR. Alterations in renal hemodynamics and function in separate kidneys during stimulation of renal artery nerves in dogs. Amer J Physiol 167: 523-530, 1951.

459. Houck CR. Effect of hydration and dehydration on hypertension in the chronic bilaterally nephrectomized dog. Amer J Physiol 176: 183-189, 1954.

460. Hsu CH, Kurtz TW, Slavicek JM. Effect of exogenous angiotensin II on renal hemodynamics in the awake rat. Circ Res 646-650, 1980.

461. Huang WC, Bell PD, Ploth DW, Navar LG. Bilateral renal function responses to converting enzyme inhibitor (SQ 20881) in one-clip, two-kidney renal hypertensive rats. Physiologist 22: 59, 1979.

462. Huber EG. Systolic blood pressure of healthy adults in relation to body weight. JAMA 88: 1554-1557, 1927.

463. Hudak WJ, Buckley JP. Production of hypertensive rats by experimental stress. J Pharmacol Sci 50: 263-264, 1961.

464. Hulthen L, Hokfelt B. The effect of converting enzyme inhibitor SQ 20881 on kinins, renin-angiotensin-aldosterone and catecholamines in relation to blood pressure in hypertensive patients. Acta Med Scand 204: 497-502, 1978.

465. Humphrey SJ, Wilson E, Zins GR. Whole body tissue

blood flow in conscious dogs treated with minoxdil. Fed Proc 33: 583, 1974.

466. Hutchins PM. Arterial rarefaction in hypertension. Bibl Anat 18: 166-168, 1979.

467. Hutchins PM, Darnell AE. Observation of a decreased number of small arterioles in spontaneously hypertensive rats. Circ Res 34(Suppl I): 161-165, 1974.

468. Ibsen H, Christensen NJ, Hollnagel H, Leth A, Kappelgaard AM, Grese J. plasma noradrenaline concentration in hypertensive and normotensive forty-year-old individuals: relationship to plasma renin concentration. Scand J Clin Lab Invest 40: 333-339, 1980.

469. Ichikawa S, Johnson JA, Stanton MW, Payne CG, Keitzer WF. Hemodynamic effects of an angiotensin II antagonist in rabbits with perinephritis hypertension. Proc Soc Exp Biol Med 155: 259-263, 1977.

470. Ikeda N, Marumo F, Shirataka M, Sato T. A model of overall regulation of body fluids. Ann Biomed Eng 7: 135-166, 1979.

471. Iriuchijima J. Sympathetic discharge rate in spontaneously hypertensive rats. Jap Heart J 14: 350-356, 1973.

472. Iriuchijima J. Arterial pressure in spontaneously hypertensive rats after high spinal cord section. Jap Circ J 40: 887-888, 1976.

473. Iriuchijima J, Numas Y, Suga H. Effect of increased age on hemodynamics of spontaneously hypertensive rats. Jap Heart J 16: 257-264, 1975.

474. Ito CS, Scher AM. Arterial baroreceptor fibers from the aortic region of the dog in the cervical vagus nerve. Circ Res 32: 442-446, 1973.

475. Ito CS, Scher AM. Reflexes from the aortic baroreceptor fibers in the cervical vagus of the cat and the dog. Circ Res 34: 51-60, 1974.

476. Ito CS, Scher AM. Regulation of arterial blood

pressure by aortic baroreceptors in the unanesthetized dog. Circ Res 42: 230-236, 1978.

477. Ito CS, Scher AM. Hypertension following denervation of aortic baroreceptors in unanesthetized dogs. Circ Res 45: 26-34, 1979.

478. Iwai J, Dahl LK, Knudsen KD. Genetic influence on the renin-angiotensin system: Low renin activities in hypertension-prone rats. Circ Res 32: 678-684, 1973.

479. Jaeger P, Ferguson RK, Brunner HR, Kirchertz EJ, Gavras H. Mechanism of blood pressure reduction by teprotide (SQ 20881) in rats. Kid Inter 13: 289-296, 1978.

480. Jaffe D, Sutherland LE, Barker D, Dahl LK. Effects of chronic excess salt ingestion: Morphological findings in kidneys of rats with different genetic susceptibilities to hypertension. Arch Pathol 90: 1-16, 1970.

481. John EJ, Lewis BA, Singer B. The sodium-retaining effect of renal nerve activity in the cat: role of angiotensin formation. Clin Sci Molec Med 51: 93-102, 1976.

482. Johnson BC, Epstein FH, Kjelsberg MO. Distributions and familial studies of blood pressure and serum cholesterol levels in a total community - Tecumseh, Michigan. J Chronic Dis 18: 147-160, 1965.

483. Johnson DC. A program to teach and demonstrate cardiovascular control through simulation. Physiologist 16: 636-643, 1973.

484. Johnson JA, Stubbs D, Keitzer WF. Role of the renin-angiotensin system in dogs with perinephritis hypertension. Proc Soc Exp Biol Med 152: 560-564, 1976.

485. Johnson MD, Malvin RL. Stimulation of renal sodium reabsorption by angiotensin II. Amer J Physiol 232: F298-F306, 1977.

486. Johnston CI, Millar JA, McGrath BP, Matthews PG. Long-term effects of captopril (SQ 14225) on blood pressure and hormone levels in essential

hypertension. Lancet 2: 493-496, 1979.

487. Jones A, Garwitz E, Mertens MS, Foster L. Aldosterone induced hypertension in rats. Physiologist 22: 64, 1979.

488. Jones DH, Hamilton CA, Reis JL. Choice of control groups in the appraisal of sympathetic nervous activity in essential hypertension. Clin Sci 57: 339-344, 1979.

489. Jones JV, Hallback M. Cardiovascular reactivity and design in rats with experimental "neurogenic hypertension". Acta Physiol Scand 102: 41-49, 1978.

490. Joosens JV, Willems J, Claessens J, Claes J, Lissens W. Sodium and hypertension. pp 91-110 in Nutrition and Cardiovascular Disease, eds F Fidanza, A Keys, G Ricci, J Somoggi. Morgagni Edizioni Scientifiche, Rome, 1971.

491. Judy WV, Watanabe AM, Henry DP, Besch HR Jr, Murphy WR, Hockel GM. Sympathetic nerve activity: Role in regulation of blood pressure in the spontaneously hypertensive rat. Circ Res 38(Suppl II): 21-29, 1976.

492. Judy WV, Watanabe AM, Murphy WR, Aprison BS, Yu PL. Sympathetic nerve activity and blood pressure in normotensive backcross rats genetically related to the spontaneously hypertensive rat. Hypertension 1: 598-604, 1979.

493. Julius S, Conway J. Hemodynamic studies in patients with borderline blood pressure elevation. Circulation 38: 282-288, 1968.

494. Julius S, Esler M. Autonomic nervous cardiovascular regulation in borderline hypertension. Amer J Cardiol 36: 685-696, 1975.

495. Julius S, Pascual AV, London R. Role of parasympathetic inhibition in the hyperkinetic type of borderline hypertension. Circulation 44: 413-418, 1971.

496. Julius S, Pascual AV, Reilly K, London R. Abnormalities of plasma volume in borderline hypertension. Arch Intern Med 127: 116-119, 1971.

497. Junqueira JF Jr, Krieger EM. Blood pressure and sleep in the rat in normotensive and in neurogenic hypertension. J Physiol 259: 725-735, 1976.

498. Kagawa CM, Cella JA, Van Arman CG. Action of new steroids in blocking effects of aldosterone and deoxycorticosterone on salt. Science 126: 1015-1016, 1957.

499. Kaloyanides GJ, DiBona GF, Raskin P. Pressure natriuresis in the isolated kidney. Amer J Physiol 220: 1660-1666, 1971.

500. Kannel W, Brand N, Skinner J, Dawber T, McNamara P. Relation of adiposity to blood pressure and development of hypertension: The Framingham study. Ann Intern Med 67: 48-59, 1967.

501. Kannel WB, Gordon T, Schwartz MH. Systolic versus diastolic blood pressure and risk of coronary heart disease: The Framingham Study. Amer J Cardiol 27: 335-346, 1971.

502. Katholi RE, Carey RM, Ayers CR, Vaughan ED Jr, Yancey MR, Morton CL. Production of sustained hypertension by chronic intrarenal norepinephrine infusion in conscious dogs. Circ Res 40(Suppl I): 118-126, 1977.

503. Katholi RE, Naftilan AJ, Oparil S. Importance of renal sympathetic tone in the development of DOCA-salt hypertension in the rat. Hypertension 2: 266-273, 1980.

504. Kawabe K, Watanbe TX, Shiono K, Sokabe H. Influences on blood pressure of renal isographs between spontaneously hypertensive and normotensive rats, utilizing the F1 hybrids. Jap Heart J 19: 886-899, 1978.

505. Kawashima K, Shiono K, Sokabe H. Variation of plasma and kidney renin activities among substrains of spontaneous hypertensive rats. Clin Exp Hyperten 2: 229-245, 1980.

506. Kempner W. Treatment of hypertensive vascular disease with rice diet. Amer J Med 4: 545-577, 1948.

507. Kezdi P, Wennemark J. Baroreceptor and sympathetic activity in experimental renal hypertension in the dog. Circulation 17: 785-790, 1958.

508. Khairallah PA, Toth A, Bumpus FM. Analogs of angiotensin II. II. Mechanism of receptor interaction. J Medicinal Chem 13: 181-184, 1970.

509. Khosla MC, Leese RA, Maloy WL, Ferreira AT, Smeby RR, Bumpus FM. Synthesis of some analogs of angiotensin II as specific antagonists of the parent hormone. J Medicinal Chem 15: 792-795, 1972.

510. Khosla MC, Page IH, Bumpus FM. Interrelations between various blood pressure regulatory systems and the mosaic theory of hypertension. Biochem Pharmacol 28: 2867-2882, 1979.

511. Kim KE, Onesti G, Del Guercio ET, Greco JG, Fernandes M, Eidelson B, Swartz C. Sequential hemodynamic changes in end-stage renal disease and the anephric state during volume expansion. Hypertension 2: 102-110, 1980.

512. Kimbrough HM Jr, Vaughan ED Jr, Carey RM, Ayers CR. Effect of intrarenal angiotensin II blockade on renal function in conscious dogs. Circ Res 40: 174-178, 1977.

513. Kirkendall WM, Connor WE, Abboud F, Rastogi SP, Anderson TA, Fry M. The effect of dietary sodium chloride on blood pressure, body fluids, electrolytes, renal function, and serum lipids of normotensive man. J Lab Clin Med 87: 418-434, 1976.

514. Kline RL, Ciriello J, Mercer PF. Effect of renal denervation on changes in arterial pressure after aortic depressor nerve transection in the rat. Fed Proc 39: 962, 1980.

515. Kline RL, Kelton PM, Mercer PF. Effect of renal denervation on the development of hypertension in spontaneously hypertensive rats. Canad J Physiol Pharmacol 56: 818-822, 1978.

516. Kline RL, Mercer PF. Functional reinnervation and development of supersensitivity to NE after renal denervation in rats. Amer J Physiol 238: R353-R358, 1980.

517. Kline RL, Mercer PF. Inhibition of angiotensin I converting enzyme prevents hypertension due to aortic depressor nerve transection in rats. Physiologist 23(4): 64, 1980.

518. Kochar MS, Itskovitz HD. Effects of hydrochlorothiazide in hypertensive patients and the need for potassium supplementation. Curr Ther Res 15: 298-304, 1973.

519. Koike H, Ito K, Miyamoto M, Nishino H. Effect of long-term blockade of angiotensin converting enzyme with captopril (SQ 14225) on hemodynamics and circulating blood volume in SHR. Hypertension 2: 299-303, 1980.

520. Kojima A, Kubota T, Sato A, Yamada T, Yamori Y, Okamoto K. Congenital abnormality of pituitary-thyroid axis in spontaneously hypertensive rats (SHR) and stroke prone rats (SPR). Pro Soc Exp Med 150: 571-573, 1975.

521. Kokubu T, Hiwada K, Shishido M, Murakami E, Hashimoto H. Reduced responses of renin release to three different stimuli in essential hypertensive patients of stage II (WHO stage classification). Clin Exp Hyperten 2: 183-196, 1980.

522. Koletsky S. Role of salt and renal mass in experimental hypertension. Arch Path 68: 11-22, 1959.

523. Koletsky S, Goodsitt AM. Natural history and pathogenesis of renal ablation hypertension. Arch Path 69: 654-662, 1960.

524. Koletsky S, Pritchard WH. Failure to demonstrate vasopressor material in salt hypertensive rats. Amer J Physiol 207: 152-154, 1964.

525. Koletsky S, Rivera-Velez JM. Renin-angiotensin system in microembolic renal hypertension. Arch Pathol 85: 1-9, 1968.

526. Kolff WJ, Page IH. Blood pressure reducing function of the kidney; reduction of renoprival hypertension by kidney perfusion. Amer J Physiol 178: 75-81, 1954.

527. Kolff WJ, Page IH, Corcoran AC. Pathogenesis of renoprival cardiovascular disease in dogs. Amer J Physiol 178: 237-245, 1954.

528. Kolloch R, Eide I, Myers M, Whigham H, DeQuattro V. Central and peripheral noradrenergic activity in renovascular hypertensive rats. Kid Inter 17: 410, 1980.

529. Komanicky P, Dale SL, Melby JC. Role of the kidney in DOCA-induced hypertension: A prolonged time-course study in the rat. Clin Res 26: 364A, 1978.

530. Komanicky P, Melby JC. Aldosterone-induced hypertension is associated with cerebromegaly in the rat. Clin Res 26: 611A, 1978.

531. Korner PI, West MJ, Shaw J, Uther JB. Steady-state properties of the baroreceptor-heart rate reflex in essential hypertension in man. Clin Exp Pharmacol Physiol 1: 65-76, 1974.

532. Kostrzewa RM, Jacobowitz DM. Pharmacological actions of 6-hydroxydopamine. Pharmacol Rev 26: 199-288, 1974.

533. Kottke FJ, Kubicek WG, Visscher MB. The production of arterial hypertension by chronic renal artery nerve stimulation. Amer J Physiol 145: 38-47, 1945.

534. Kovach JC. Extracellular fluid volume in hypertension. Canad Med Ass J 75: 934-935, 1956.

535. Krakoff LR, Goodwin FJ, Baer L, Torres M, Laragh JH. The role of renin in the exaggerated natriuresis of hypertension. Circulation 42: 335-345, 1970.

536. Krakoff LR, Selvadurai R, Sutter E. Effect of methylprednisolone upon arterial pressure and the renin angiotensin system in the rat. Amer J Physiol 228: 613-617, 1975.

537. Kramer P, Ochwadt B. Sodium excretion in Goldblatt hypertension. Pflugers Arch 332: 332-345, 1972.

538. Krieger EM. Neurogenic hypertension in the rat. Circ Res 15: 511-521, 1964.

539. Krieger EM. Time course of baroreceptor resetting in acute hypertension. Amer J Physiol 218: 486-490, 1970.

540. Krieger EM, Brenes JR, Salgado HC, Assan CJ, Salgado MCO. Role of the baroreceptor reflex in the early phases after removing the renal artery constriction in conscious renal hypertensive rats. Acta Physiol Latinoamer 27: 49-58, 1977.

541. Krieger EM, Moreira ED, Silveira LF. Hemodynamic studies in conscious neurogenic hypertensive rats. Jap Heart J 20(Suppl I): 68-70, 1979.

542. Krieger EM, Salgado HC, Assan HC, Greene LLJ, Ferreira SH. Potential screening test for detection of overactivity of renin-angiotensin system. Lancet 1: 269-271, 1971.

543. Krista LM, Waibel PE, Shoffner RN, Sautter JH. Natural dissecting aneurysm (aortic rupture) and blood pressure in the turkey. Nature 214: 1162-1163, 1967.

544. Kubicek Wg, Kottke FJ, Laker DJ, Visscher MB. Renal function during arterial hypertension produced by chronic splanchnic nerve stimulation in the dog. Amer J Physiol 174: 397-400, 1953.

545. Kubo T, Hashimoto M. Effects of intraventricular and intraspinal 6-hydroxydopamine on blood pressure of spontaneously hypertensive rats. Arch Inter Pharmacodyn 232: 166-176, 1978.

546. Kubo T, Hashimoto M. Effects of intraventricular and intraspinal 6-hydroxydopamine in blood pressure of DOCA-saline hypertensive rats. Arch Inter Pharmacodyn 238: 50-59, 1979.

547. Kubo T, Hashimoto M, Ohashi T. Effects of intraventricular and intraspinal 6-hydroxydopamine on blood pressure of renal hypertensive rats. Arch Inter Pharmacodyn 234: 270-278, 1978.

548. Kumamoto K, Yamamoto Y, Kawasaki T, Omae T, Tanaka K. Effect of acute volume depletion on blood pressure, plasma renin activity and plasma aldosterone concentration in hypertensive subjects. Jap Circ J 39: 545-549, 1975.

549. Kumar D, Hall AED, Nakashima R, Gornall AG. Studies on aldosterone. II. Hypertension as a cumulative effect of aldosterone administration. Canad J Biochem Physiol 35: 113-118, 1957.

550. Kunes J, Capek K, Jelinek J, Cherkovich GM. Extracellular fluid distribution in salt-hypertensive monkeys. Experientia 34: 753-754, 1978.

551. Kunes J, Jelinek J. Extracellular fluid distribution in rats with chronic one- and two-kidney Goldblatt hypertension. Clin Exp Pharmacol Physiol 6: 507-513, 1979.

552. Kurihara H, Tanaka T, Terasawa F, Seki M, Ikeda M. Difference in changes of plasma volume in two types of Goldblatt hypertension in rabbits. Tohoku J Exp Med 118: 113-125, 1976.

553. Lack A, Aldolph W, Ralston W, Leiby G, Winsor T, Griffith G. Biomicroscopy of conjunctional vessels in hypertension. Amer Heart J 38: 654-664, 1949.

554. Lais LT, Shaffer RA, Brody MJ. Neurogenic and humoral factors controlling vascular resistance in the spontaneously hypertensive rat. Circ Res 35: 764-774, 1974.

555. Lake CR, Ziegler MG, Coleman MD, Kopin IJ. Age-adjusted plasma norepinephrine levels are simular in normotensive and hypertensive subjects. New Eng J Med 296: 208-209, 1977.

556. Laks MM, Garner D, Wong V. Increased ejection fraction produced by a long-term subhypertensive infusion of norepinephrine in the conscious dog. Amer Heart J 98: 732-735, 1979.

557. Lamprecht F, Richardson JS, Williams RB, Kopin IJ. 6-hydroxydopamine destruction of central adrenergic neurones prevents or reverses developing DOCA-salt hypertension in rats. J Neural Transmission 40: 149-158, 1977.

558. Langford HG, Watson RL. Electrolytes and hypertension. pp 119-128 in Epidemiology of Hypertension, ed PO Stratton. Intercontinental Medical Book Co, New York, 1974.

559. Langston JB, Guyton AC, Douglas BH, Dorsett PE. Effect of changes in salt intake on arterial pressure and renal function in partially nephrectomized dogs. Circ Res 12: 508-513, 1963.

560. Laragh JH, Baer L, Brunner HR, Buhler FR, Sealey JE, Vaughan ED Jr. Renin, angiotensin and aldosterone system in pathogenesis and management of hypertensive vascular disease. Amer J Med 52: 633-652, 1972.

561. Laragh JH, Case DB, Atlas SA, Sealy JE. Captopril compared with other antirenin system agents in hypertensive patients: Its triphasic effects on blood pressure and its use to identify and treat the renin factor. Hypertension 2: 586-593, 1980.

562. Laubie M, Schmitt H. Destruction of the nucleus tractus solitarii in the dog: Comparison with sinoaortic denervation. Amer J Physiol 236: H736-H743, 1979.

563. Laycock JF, Penn W, Shirley DG, Walter SJ. The role of vasopressin in blood pressure regulation immediately following acute hemorrhage in the rat. J Physiol 296: 267-275, 1979.

564. Ledingham JM, Cohen RD. Circulatory changes during the reversal of experimental hypertension. Clin Sci 22: 69-77, 1962.

565. Ledingham JM, Cohen RD. Hypertension explained by Starling's theory of circulatory homeostasis. Lancet 1: 887, 1963.

566. Ledingham JM, Pelling D. Cardiac output and peripheral resistance in experimental renal hypertension. Circ Res 21(Suppl II): 187-199, 1967.

567. Ledingham JM, Pelling D. Hemodynamic and other studies in the renoprival hypertensive rat. J Physiol 210: 233-253, 1970.

568. Lee DR, Simpson FO. Effect of propranolol on blood pressure, heart rate and exchangeable sodium in genetically hypertensive and normotensive rats. Proc Univ Otago Med Sch 51: 51-52, 1973.

569. Lee DR, Simpson FO. Effect of propranolol on plasma volume and renin levels of genetically hypertensive

rats. Proc Univ Otago Med Sch 51: 53-54, 1973.

570. Lee RE, Holze EA. Peripheral vascular hemodynamics in the bulbar conjunctiva of subjects with hypertensive vascular disease. J Clin Invest 30: 539-546, 1951.

571. Leenen FHH, de Jong W. A solid silver clip for induction of predictable levels of renal hypertension in the rat. J Appl Physiol 31: 142-144, 1971.

572. Leenen FHH, Scheeren JW, Omylanowski D, Elema JD, Van Der Wal B, de Jong W. Changes in the renin-angiotensin-aldostrone system and in sodium and potassium balance during development of renal hypertension in rats. Clin Sci Molec Med 48: 17-26, 1975.

573. Leishman AWD. Hypertension-treated and untreated: A study of 400 cases. Brit Med J 1: 1361-1368, 1959.

574. Lenel R, Katz LN, Rodbard S. Arterial hypertension in the chicken. Amer J Physiol 152: 557-562, 1948.

575. Leonards JR, Heisler CR. Blood pressure of bilaterally nephrectomized dogs. Fed Proc 11: 247, 1952.

576. Leslie BR, Case DB, Sullivan JF, Vaughan ED Jr. Absence of blood-pressure lowering effect of captopril in anephric patients. Brit Med J 1: 1067-1068, 1980.

577. Levinsky NG. Natriuretic hormones. Advances Metab Dis 7: 37-71, 1974.

578. Levy RL, Hillman CC, Stroud WD, White PD. Transient hypertension: Its significance in terms of later development of sustained hypertension and cardiovascular-renal diseases. JAMA 126: 829-833, 1944.

579. Levy RL, White PD, Stroud WD, Hillman CC. Overweight: Its prognostic significance in relation to hypertension and cardiovascular-renal diseases. JAMA 131: 951-953, 1946.

580. Lew EA. Blood pressure and mortality: Life insurance experience. pp 392-396 in <u>The Epidemiology</u>

of Hypertension, eds J Stamler, R Stamler, TN Pullman. Grune and Stratton, New York, 1967.

581. Lewis PJ, Haeusler G. Reduction in sympathetic nervous activity as a mechanism for hypotensive effect of propranolol. Nature 256: 440, 1975.

582. Lewis PJ, Lee MR. Plasma renin activity in the rabbit with renal hypertension. Brit J Exp Pathol 52: 478-481, 1971.

583. Liard JF. Effet de l'ablation partielle ou totale du tissu renal sur l'hypertension renovasculaire chez le rat. Experientia 25: 934-935, 1969.

584. Liard JF. Sodium retention versus renin-angiotensin system in experimental renal hypertension. Canad J Physiol 51: 238-241, 1973.

585. Liard JF. Hemodynamics and body fluid volumes in response to fluid loading in conscious dogs: non-excretory renal influences. Clin Sci Molec Med 51: 243-255, 1976.

586. Liard JF. Renal denervation delays blood pressure increase in the spontaneously hypertensive rat. Experientia 33: 339-340. 1977.

587. Liard JF. Hypertension induced by prolonged intracoronary administration of dobutamine in conscious dogs. Clin Sci Molec Med 54: 153-160, 1978.

588. Liard JF. Cardiogenic hypertension: experimental evidence from a comparison between intravenous and intracoronary administration of dobutamine in conscious dogs. Clin Sci 58: 271-277, 1980.

589. Liard JF. Changes in cardiac output and skeletal muscle blood flow in dogs with salt-loading hypertension. Experientia 36: 698, 1980.

590. Liard JF, Cowley AW Jr, McCaa RE, McCaa CS, Guyton AC. Renin, aldosterone, body fluid volumes, and the baroreceptor reflex in the development and reversal of Goldblatt hypertension in conscious dogs. Circ Res 34: 549-560, 1974.

591. Liard JF, Peters G. Mechanism of the fall in blood

pressure after 'unclamping' in rats with Goldblatt-type hypertension . Experientia 26: 743-745, 1970.

592. Liddle GW, Sennett JA. New mineralocorticoids in the syndrome of low-renin essential hypertension. J Ster Biochem 6: 751-753, 1975.

593. Lippert H, Lehmann HP. SI Units in Medicine. Urban and Schwarzenberg, Baltimore-Munich, 1978.

594. Littler WA, Honour AJ, Sleight P, Stott FD. Continuous recording of direct arterial pressure and electrocardiogram in unrestricted man. Brit Med J 3: 76-78, 1972.

595. Liu K, Cooper R, McKeever J, McKeever P, Byington R, Soltero I, Stamler R, Gosch F, Stevens E, Stamler J. Assessment of the association between habitual salt intake and high blood pressure: Methodological problems. Amer J Epidem 110: 219-226, 1979.

596. Liu K, Dyer AR, Cooper RS, Stamler R, Stamler J. Can 24-hour urine collection be replaced by overnight urine for assessment of salt intake? Hypertension 1: 529-536, 1979.

597. Lohmeier TE, Cowley AW Jr. Hypertensive and renal effects of chronic low-level intrarenal angiotensin infusion in the dog. Circ Res 44: 154-160, 1979.

598. Lohmeier TE, Cowley AW Jr, DeClue JW, Guyton AC. Failure of chronic aldosterone infusion to increase arterial pressure in dogs with angiotensin-induced hypertension. Circ Res 43: 381-390, 1978.

599. London GM, Safar ME, Weiss YA, Simon AC. Total effective compliance of the vascular bed in essential hypertension. Amer Heart J 95: 325-330, 1978.

600. Louis WJ, Doyle AE, Anavekar SN. Plasma noradrenaline concentration and blood pressure in essential hypertension, phaeochromocytoma and depression. Clin Sci Molec Med 48(Suppl II): 239s-242s, 1975.

601. Louis WJ, Doyle AE, Anaveker SN, Chua KG. Sympathetic activity and essential hypertension. Clin Sci Molec Med 45(Suppl): 119s-121s, 1973.

602. Louis WJ, Tabei R, Spector S. Effects of sodium intake on inherited hypertension in the rat. Lancet 2: 1283-1286, 1971.

603. Lowenstein J, Beranbaum ER, Chasis H, Baldwin DS. Intrarenal pressure and exaggerated natriuresis in essential hypertension. Clin Sci 38: 359-374, 1970.

604. Lucas J, Floyer MA. Body fluid distribution and pressure in experimental hypertension. Clin Sci 42: 2P, 1972.

605. Lucas J, Floyer MA. Renal control of changes in the compliance of the interstitial space: A factor in the etiology of renoprival hypertension. Clin Sci 44: 397-416, 1973.

606. Luetscher JA Jr, Johnson BB. Observations on the sodium-retaining corticoid (aldosterone) in the urine of children and adults in relation to sodium balance and edema. J Clin Invest 23: 1441-1446, 1954.

607. Luft FC, Rankin LI, Henry DP, Bloch R, Grim CE, Weyman AE, Murray RH, Weinberger MH. Plasma and urinary norepinephrine values at extremes of sodium intake in normal man. Hypertension 1: 261-266, 1979.

608. Lund-Johanson P. Hemodynamic long-term effects of timolol at rest and during exercise in essential hypertension. Acta Med Scand 199: 263-267, 1976.

609. Lundin H, Mark R. Feeding of protein to partially nephrectomized animals. J Metab Res 7-8: 221-257, 1925.

610. Lupu AN, Maxwell MH, Kaufman JJ. Mechanisms of hypertension during the chronic phase of the one-clip, two-kidney model in the dog. Circ Res 40 (Suppl I): 57-61, 1977.

611. Lupu AN, Maxwell MH, Kaufman JJ, White FN. Experimental unilateral renal artery constriction in the dog. Circ Res 30: 567-574, 1972.

612. Macdonald GJ, Boyd GW, Peart WS. Effect of the angiotensin II blocker 1-Sar,8-Ala Angiotensin II on renal artery clip hypertension in the rat. Circ Res 37: 640-646, 1975.

613. Man in't Veld AJ, Schicht IM, Derkx HM, deBruyn JHB, Schalekamp MADH. Effects of an angiotensin-converting enzyme inhibitor (captopril) on blood pressure in anephric subjects. Brit Med J 1: 288-290, 1980.

614. Mancia G, Ludbrook J, Ferrrari A, Gregorini L, Zanchetti A. Baroreceptor reflexes in human hypertension. Circ Res 43: 170-177, 1978.

615. Manger WM, Gifford RW Jr. Pheochromocytoma. Springer-Verlag, New York, 1977.

616. Manning RD Jr. Lack of nonexcretory renal influences on hemodynamics and fluid volume distribution after the volume loading of conscious dogs. Circ Res 46: 880-886, 1980.

617. Manning RD Jr, Coleman TG, Guyton AC, Norman RA Jr, McCaa RE. Essential role of mean circulatory filling pressure in salt-induced hypertension. Amer J Physiol 236: R40-R47, 1979.

618. Manning RD Jr, Guyton AC, Coleman TG, McCaa RE. Hypertension in dogs during antidiuretic hormone and hypotonic saline infusion. Amer J Physiol 236: H314-H322, 1979.

619. Manthorpe T. Antihypertensive and hypertensive effects of the kidney. Acta Pathol Microbiol Scand Sect A 83: 395-405, 1975.

620. Markiewicz A, Wojezuk D, Kokot F, Cicha A. Plasma renin activity in coarctation of aorta before and after surgery. Brit Heart J 37: 721-725, 1975.

621. Marks ES, Bing RF, Thurston H, Swales JD. Vasopressor property of the converting enzyme inhibitor captopril (SQ 14225): The role of factors other than renin-angiotensin blockade in the rat. Clin Sci 58: 1-6, 1980.

622. Marks LS, Maxwell MH. Tigerstedt and the discovery of renin. Hypertension 1: 384-388, 1979.

623. Marshall GR. Structure-activity relations of antagonists of the renin- angiotensin system. Fed Proc 35: 2494-2501, 1976.

624. Martin L. Effect of weight reduction on normal and raised blood pressures in obesity. Lancet 2: 1051-1053, 1952.

625. Masaki Z, Ferrario CM, Bumpus FM. Effects of SQ 20,881 on the intact kidney of dogs with two-kidney, one clip hypertension. Hypertension 2: 649-656, 1980.

626. Master AM, Garfield CI, Walters MB. Normal Blood Pressure and Hypertension. Lea and Febiger, Philadelphia, 1952.

627. Master AM, Marks HH, Dacks S. Hypertension in people over 40. JAMA 121: 1251-1256, 1943.

628. Mathias CJ, Christensen NJ, Corbett JL, Frankel HL, Spalding JMK. Plasma catecholamines during paroxysmal neurogenic hypertension in quadriplegic man. Circ Res 39: 204-208, 1976.

629. Matthews PG, Johnson CI. Augmented circulating bradykinin following angiotensin converting enzyme inhibition. Exp Pharmacol Physiol 7: 62-63, 1980.

630. Maxwell MH, Lupu AN, Viskoper RJ, Arabena LA, Waks VA. Mechanisms of hypertension during the acute and intermediate phases of the one-clip, two-kidney model in the dogs. Circ Res 40(suppi I): 24-28, 1977.

631. McAllister RG Jr, Michelakis AM, Oates JA, Foster JH. Malignant hypertension due to renal artery stenosis: Greater renin release from the nonstenotic kidney. JAMA 221: 865-868, 1972.

632. McCabe RE, Gomez J, Zintel HA. The production of hypertension in dogs by a single transient anoxic episode. Angiology 20: 231-242, 1969.

633. McCubbin JW. Carotid sinus participation in experimental renal hypertension. Circulation 17: 791-797, 1958.

634. McCubbin JW, DeMoura RS, Page IH, Olmsted F. Arterial hypertension elicited by subpressor amounts of angiotensin. Science 149: 1394-1395, 1965.

635. McDonald SJ, de Wardener HE. The relationship between the renal arterial perfusion pressure and the

increase in sodium excretion which occurs during an infusion of saline. Nephron 2: 1-14, 1965.

636. McDonough J, Wilhelmj CM. The effect of excessive salt intake on human blood pressure. Amer J Dig Dis 21: 180-181, 1954.

637. McIhany ML, Schaffer JW, Hines EA. The heritability of blood pressure: An investigation of 200 twin pairs using the cold pressor test. Johns Hopkins Med J 136: 57-64, 1975.

638. McNay JL, Abe Y. Pressure-dependent heterogeneity of renal cortical blood flow in dogs. Circ Res 27: 571-587, 1970.

639. McQuarrie I, Thompson WH, Anderson JA. Effects of excessive ingestion of sodium and potassium salts on carbohydrate metabolism and blood pressure in diabetic children. J Nutr 11: 77-101, 1936.

640. Melby JC, Dale SL. Adrenal steroidogensis in "low-renin" or hyporeninemic hypertension. J Ster Biochem 6: 761-766, 1975.

641. Meneely GR, Ball COT, Youmans JB. Chronic sodium chloride toxicity: Protective effect of added potassium chloride. Ann Intern Med 47: 263-273, 1957.

642. Meneely GR, Battarbee HD. Sodium and potassium. Nutr Rev 34: 225-235, 1976.

643. Meneely GR, Tucker RG, Darby WJ, Huerback SH. Sodium chloride toxicity in the albino rat. J Exp Med 98: 71-80, 1953.

644. Merrill JP, Giordano C, Heetderks DR. The role of the kidney in human hypertension. I. Failure of hypertension to develop in the renoprival subject. Amer J Med 31: 931-940, 1961.

645. Meyer P, Worcel M. Role of angiotensin of in the salt hypertension of rats. Pflueger Arch 317: 327-335, 1970.

646. Miall WE. Follow-up study of arterial pressure in the population of a Welsh mining valley. Brit Med J 2: 1204-1210, 1959.

647. Miall WE, Heneage P, Khosla T, Lovell HG, Moore F. Factors influencing the degree of resemblance in arterial pressure of close relatives. Clin Sci 33: 271-283, 1967.

648. Michael VF, Mukherjee SK, Meeks LA. Acute effects of furosemide in the functionally anephric, normovolemic, spontaneously hypertensive rat. Clin Res 28: 18A, 1980.

649. Michelakis AM, McAllister RG. The effect of chronic adrenergic receptor blockade on plasma renin activity in man. J Clin Endocrinol 34: 386-394, 1972.

650. Miksche LW, Miksche U, Gross F. Effect of sodium restriction on renal hypertension and on renin activity in the rat. Circ Res 27: 973-984, 1970.

651. Miller AW II, Bohr DF, Schork AM, Terris JM. Hemodynamic responses to DOCA in young pigs. Hypertension 1: 591-597, 1979.

652. Miller ED Jr, Samuels AI, Haber E, Barger AC. Inhibition of angiotensin conversion in experimental renal hypertension. Science 177: 1108-1109, 1972.

653. Miller ED Jr, Samuels AI, Haber E, Barger AC. Inhibition of angiotensin conversion and prevention of renal hypertension. Amer J Physiol 228: 448-453, 1975.

654. Miller HC, Phillips CE. Subsequent nephrectomy of the contralateral kidney for recurrent renovascular hypertension. Surg Obstet Gynec 127: 1274-1280, 1968.

655. Mohring J, Kintz J, Schoun J. Studies on the role of vasopressin in blood pressure control of spontaneously hypertensive rats with established hypertension (SHR, Stroke-prone strain). J Cardiovasc Pharmacol 1: 593-608, 1979.

656. Mohring J, Mohring B, Naumann HJ, Philippi A, Homsy E, Ortu H, Dauda G, Kazda S, Gross F. Salt and water balance and renin activity in renal hypertension of rats. Amer J Physiol 228: 1847-1855, 1975.

657. Mohring J, Mohring B, Petri M, Haack D. Vasopressor role of ADH in the pathogenesis of malignant DOC

hypertension. Amer J Physiol 232: F260-F269, 1977.

658. Mohring J, Mohring B, Petri M, Haack D. Plasma vasopressin concentrations and effects of vasopressin antiserum on blood pressure in rats with malignant two-kidney Goldblatt hypertension. Circ Res 42: 17-22, 1978.

659. Mohring J, Petri M, Szokol M, Haack D, Mohring B. Effects of saline drinking on malignant course of renal hypertension in rats. Amer J Physiol 230: 849-857, 1976.

660. Montgomery JC, McGregor DD. Blood pressure responses to stimulation of spinal sympathetic outflow in genetically hypertensive rats. Proc Univ Otago Med Sch 52: 36-38, 1975.

661. Moore S, Mersereau WA. Microembolic renal ischemia, hypertension, and nephrosclerosis. Arch Pathol 85: 623-630, 1968.

662. Morgan T, Adam W, Gillies A, Wilson M, Morgan G, Carney S. Hypertension treated by salt restriction. Lancet 1: 227-230, 1978.

663. Morganti A, Pickering TG, Lopez-Ovejero JA, Laragh JH. Contrasting effects of acute beta blockade with propranolol on plasma catecholamines and renin in essential hypertension: a possible basis for the delayed antihypertensive response. Amer Heart J 98: 490-494, 1979.

664. Mortimer RH, Gordon RD, Nielson GH. Relationships between blood pressure, plasma volume and plasma renin activity in coarctation of the aorta. Aust New Zeal J Med 3: 431-432, 1973.

665. Moser M. The effect of high salt intake on the treatment of hypertension. pp 512-517 in <u>Hypertension</u>, ed JH Moyer. Saunders, Philadelphia, 1959.

666. Moses C. Development of atherosclerosis in dogs with hypercholesterolemia and chronic hypertension. Circ Res 2: 243-247, 1954.

667. Moses L, Daniels GE, Nickerson JL. Psychogenic factors in essential hypertension: Methodology and

preliminary report. Psychosom Med 18: 471-485, 1956.

668. Mourant AJ. Determinants of high blood pressure in salt deprived renal hypertensive rats: Role of changes in plasma volume, extracellular fluid volume, and plasma angiotensin II. Clin Sci Molec Med 55: 81-87, 1978.

669. Muirhead EE. Case for a renomedullary blood pressure lowering hormone. Contr Nephrol 12: 69-81, 1978.

670. Muirhead EE. Antihypertensive functions of the kidney. Arthur C. Corcoran Memorial Lecture. Hypertension 2: 444-464, 1980.

671. Muirhead EE, Brooks B. Reversal of one-kidney, one-clip hypertension by unclipping: The renal, sodium-volume relationship reexamined. Proc Soc Exp Med Biol 163: 540-546, 1980.

672. Muirhead EE, Brooks B, Brosius WL. Renomedullary deficiency: A permissive factor in renoprival hypertension. Arch Path 95: 77-80, 1973.

673. Muirhead EE, Brooks B, Pitcock JA, Stephenson P. Renomedullary antihypertensive function in accelerated (malignant) hypertension. J Clin Invest 51: 181-190, 1972.

674. Muirhead EE, Brooks B, Pitcock JA, Stephenson P, Brosius WL. Role of the renal medulla in the sodium-sensitive component of renoprival hypertension. Lab Invest 27: 192-198, 1972.

675. Muirhead EE, Jones F, Graham P. Hypertension in bilaterally nephrectomized dogs in absence of exogenous sodium excess. Arch Pathol 56: 286-292, 1953.

676. Muirhead EE, Jones F, Stirman J. Hypertensive cardiovascular disease of dog. Relation of sodium and dietary protein to ureterocaval anastomosis and ureteral ligation. Arch Pathol 70: 108-116, 1960.

677. Muirhead EE, Leach BE, Armstrong FB. Angiotension-salt hypertension. Clin Sci Molec Med 45(Suppl): 257s-261s, 1973.

678. Muirhead EE, Rightsel WA, Leach BE, Byers LW, Pitcock JA, Brooks B. Reversal of hypertension by transplants and lipid extracts of cultured renomedullary interstitial cells. Lab Invest 35: 162-172,1977.

679. Muirhead EE, Stirman JA, Jones F. Renal autoexplantation and a functional characterization of nonexcretory renal tissue. J Clin Invest 38: 1027-1028, 1959.

680. Muirhead EE, Stirman JA, Lesch W, Jones F. The reduction of postnephrectomy hypertension by renal homotransplant. Surg Gynec Obstet 103: 673-686, 1956.

681. Muller JM, Schlittler E, Bein HJ. Reserpin, der sedative Wirkstoff aus Rauwolfia serpentina Benth. Experientia 8: 338, 1952.

682. Munoz-Ramirez H, Chatelain RE, Bumpus FM, Khairallah PA. Development of two-kidney Goldblatt hypertension in rats under dietary sodium restriction. Amer J Physiol 238: H889-H894, 1980.

683. Murphy RJF. Effect of "rice diet" on plasma volume and extracellular fluid space in hypertensive subjects. J Clin Invest 29: 912-917, 1950.

684. Murphy WR, Coleman TG. The effects of antihypertensive drug treatments on rats with aortic coarctation. Fed Proc 38: 883, 1979.

685. Murray RH, Luft FC, Bloch R, Weyman AE. Blood response to extremes of sodium intake in normal man. Proc Soc Exp Biol Med 159: 432-436, 1978.

686. Murthy VS, Waldron TL, Goldberg ME. The mechanism of bradykinin potentiation after inhibition of angiotensin-converting enzyme by SQ 14225 in conscious rabbits. Circ Res 43(Suppl I): 40-45, 1978.

687. Murthy VS, Waldron TL, Goldberg ME, Vollmer RR. Inhibition of angiotensin converting enzyme by SQ 14225 in conscious rabbits. Europ J Pharmacol 46: 207-212, 1977.

688. Nagatsu T, Kato T, Numata Y, Ikuta K, Umezawa H,

Tokeuchi T. Serum dopamine beta-hydroxylase activity in developing spontaneously hypertensive rats and the effect of salt adimintration. Jap Heart J 16: 324-325, 1975.

689. Nathan MA, Reis DJ. Chronic labile hypertension production by lesions of the nucleus tractus solitarii in the cat. Circ Res 40: 72-81, 1977.

690. Navar LG, LaGrange RA, Bell PD, Thomas CE, Ploth DW. Glomerular and renal hemodynamics during converting enzyme inhibition (SQ 14225) in the dog. Hypertension 1: 371-377, 1979.

691. Nestel PJ. Blood pressure and catecholamines excretion after mental stress in labile hypertension. Lancet 1: 692-694, 1969.

692. Ng KKF, Vane JR. Fate of angiotensin I in the circulation. Nature 218: 144-150, 1968.

693. Nicholls MG, Kiowski W, Zweifler AJ, Julius S, Schork MA, Greenhouse JG. Plasma norepinephrine variations with dietary sodium intake. Hypertension 2: 29-32, 1980.

694. Nicholls MG, Ramsay LE, Boddy K, Fraser R, Morton JJ, Robertson JIS. Mineralocorticoid-induced blood pressure, electrolyte, and hormone changes, and reversal with spironolactone, in healthy men. Metabolism 28: 584-593, 1979.

695. Nies A, Robinson DS, Lamborn KR, Lampert RP. Genetic control of platelet and plasma monoamine oxidase activity. Arch Gen Psychiat 28: 834-838, 1973.

696. Nolla-Panades J. Hypertension and increased hindlimb vascular reactivity in experimental coarctation of the aorta. Circ Res 12: 3-9, 1963.

697. Noordergraaf A. Hemodynamics. pp 391-545 in Biological Engineering, ed HP Schwan. McGraw-Hill, New York, 1969.

698. Noresson E, Ricksten SE, Thoren P. Left atrial pressure in normotensive and spontaneously hypertensive rats. Acta Physiol Scand 107: 9-12, 1979.

699. Norman RA Jr, Coleman TG. Potential errors in arterial pressure measurement in restrained rats. Fed Proc 39:973 1980.

700. Norman RA Jr, Coleman TG, Wiley TL Jr, Manning RD Jr, Guyton AC. The separate roles of sodium ion concentration and fluid volumes in salt-loading hypertension in sheep. Amer J Physiol 229: 1068-1072, 1975.

701. Norman RA Jr, Enobakhare JA, DeClue JW, Douglas BH, Guyton AC. Arterial pressure - urinary output relationship in hypertensive rats. Amer J Physiol 234: R98-R103, 1978.

702. Nosaka S, Wang SC. Carotid sinus baroreceptor functions in the spontaneously hypertensive rat. Amer J Physiol 222: 1079-1084, 1972.

703. Nowak SJG. Chronic hypertension produced by carotid sinus and aortic-depressor nerve section. Ann Surg 3: 102-111, 1940.

704. Numas Y, Suga H, Iriuchijima J. Cardiac output in conscious SHR. Jap Heart J 16: 338-339, 1975.

705. Oates HF, Stokes GS, Storey BG. Plasma renin concentration in hypertension produced by unilateral renal artery constriction in the rat. Clin Exp Pharmacol Physiol 2: 289-296, 1975.

706. Oates JA, Gillespie L, Udenfriend S, Sjoerdsma. Decarboxylase inhibition and blood pressure reduction by alpha-methyl-3,4-dihydroxy-DL-phenylalanine. Science 131: 1890-1891, 1960.

707. Oelkers W, Schoneshofer M, Schultze G, Bauer B. Effect of prolonged low dose infusions of Ile-5 angiotensin II on blood pressure, aldosterone and electrolyte excretion in sodium replete man. Klin Wschr 56: 37-41, 1978.

708. Ogden E, Page EW, Anderson E. Effect of posterior hypophysectomy on renal hypertension. Amer J Physiol 141: 389-392, 1944.

709. Okamoto K. _Spontaneous Hypertension : Its Pathogenesis and Complications_. Springer-Verlag, Berlin, 1972.

710. Okamoto K, Aoki K. Development of a strain of spontaneously hypertensive rats. Jap Circ J 27: 282-293, 1963.

711. Oliver G, Schafer EA. On the physiological action of extracts of pituitary body and certain other glandular organs. J Physiol 18: 277-279, 1895.

712. Oliver WJ, Cohen EL, Neel JV. Blood pressure, sodium intake, and sodium related hormones in the Yanomamo Indians, a "no-salt" culture. Circulation 52: 146-151, 1975.

713. Olmsted F, Page IH. Hemodynamic aspects of prolonged infusion of angiotensin into unanesthesized dogs. Circ Res 16: 140-149, 1965.

714. Olmsted F, Page IH. Hemodynamic changes in trained dogs during experimental renal hypertension. Circ Res 16: 134-139, 1965.

715. Omvik P, Tarazi RC, Bravo EL. Regulation of sodium balance in hypertension. Hypertension 2: 515-523, 1980.

716. Ondetti MA, Rubin B, Cushman DW. Design of specific inhibitors of angiotensin-converting enzyme: New class of orally active antihypertensive agents. Science 196: 441-444, 1977.

717. Ondetti MA, Williams NJ, Sabo EF, Pluscec J, Weaver ER, Kocy O. Angiotensin-converting enzyme inhibitors from the venom of <u>Bothrops jararaca</u>. Isolation, elucidation of structure, and synthesis. Biochemistry 10: 4033-4039, 1971.

718. Onesti G, Kim KE, Greco JA, del Guercio ET, Fernandes M, Swartz C. Blood pressure regulation in end-stage renal disease and anephric man. Circ Res 36(Suppl I): 145-152, 1975.

719. Onesti G, Swartz C, Ramirez O, Brest AN. Bilaterally nephrectomy for control of hypertension in uremia. Trans Amer Soc Artif Intern Organs 14: 361-364, 1968.

720. Onoyama K, Bravo EL, Tarazi RC. Sodium, extracellular fluid volumes, and cardiac output changes in the genesis of mineralocorticoid

hypertension in the intact dog. Hypertension 1: 331-336, 1979.

721. Oparil S, Erinoff L, Cutilletta A. Catecholamines, blood pressure, renin and myocardial function in the spontaneously hypertensive rat. Clin Sci Molec Med 51: 455s-459s, 1976.

722. Orbison JL, Christian CL, Peters E. Studies on experimental hypertension and cardiovascular disease. I. A method for production of malignant hypertension in bilaterally nephrectomized dogs. Arch Path 54: 185-196, 1952.

723. Otsuka Y, Carretero OA, Albertini R, Binia A. Angiotensin and sodium balance: Their role in chronic two-kidney Goldblatt hypertension. Hypertension 1: 389-396, 1979.

724. Overbeck HW. Hemodynamics of early experimental renal hypertension in dogs. Circ Res 31: 653-663, 1972.

725. Overbeck HW. Cardiovascular hypertrophy and "waterlogging" in coarctation hypertension. Hypertension 1: 486-492, 1979.

726. Overbeck HW. The sodium pump in cardiovascular muscle in hypertension: Whose hypothesis? Clin Exp Hyperten 1: 551-556, 1979.

727. Overbeck HW, Molnar JI, Haddy FJ. Resistance to blood flow through the vascular bed of the dog forelimb. Amer J Card 8: 533-541, 1961.

728. Padfield PL, Brown JJ, Lever AF, Morton JJ, Robertson JIS. Changes of vasopressin in hypertension: Cause or effect? Lancet 1: 1255-1257, 1976.

729. Page IH. The production of persistent arterial hypertension by cellophane perinephritis. JAMA 113: 2046-2048, 1939.

730. Page IH. Pathogenesis of arterial hypertension. JAMA 140: 451-457, 1949.

731. Page IH. The discovery of angiotensin. Persp Biol Med 18: 456-462, 1975.

732. Page IH, Dustan HP. A new, potent antihypertensive drug : Preliminary study of (2'-(octahydro-1-azocinyl)-ethyl) - guanidine sulfate (guanethidine). JAMA 170: 1265-1271, 1959.

733. Page IH, Helmer OM. A crystalline pressor substance (angiotonin) resulting from the reaction between renin and renin activator. J Exp Med 71: 29-42, 1940.

734. Page IH, Lewis LA. Influence of protein, carbohydrate and salt on arterial pressure of dogs with experimental renal hypertension. Amer J Physiol 156: 422-428, 1949.

735. Page IH, Oparil S, Bohr DF, Tobian L. Nomenclature for experimental renovascular hypertension. Hypertension 1: 61, 1979.

736. Page IH, Sweet JE. The effect of hypophysectomy of arterial blood pressure of dogs with experimental hypertension. Amer J Physiol 120: 238-245, 1937.

737. Page LB, Damon A, Moellering RC Jr. Antecedents of cariovascular disease in six Solomon Island societies. Circulation 49: 1132-1146, 1974.

738. Pals DT, Masucci FD, Denning GS Jr, Sipos F, Fessler DC. Role of the pressor action of angiotensin II in experimental hypertension. Circ Res 29: 673-681, 1971.

739. Pamnani MB, Overbeck HW. Abnormal ion and water composition of veins and normotensive arteries in coarctation hypertension in rats. Circ Res 38: 375-378, 1976.

740. Pamnani MB, Simon G, Overbeck HW. Bioassay in vivo for circulating vasoactive agents after renal artery constriction in dogs. Circ Res 39: 517-523, 1976.

741. Pan YJ, Young DB. Experimental aldosterone hypertension. Fed Proc 37: 634, 1978.

742. Parijs J, Joosens JV, Linden LV, Verstreken G, Amery AKPC. Moderate sodium restriction and diuretics in the treatment of hypertension. Amer Heart J 85: 22-34, 1973.

743. Parker JC. Hypertension and the red cell. New Eng J Med 302: 804-805, 1980.

744. Parving H, Gyntelberg F. Transcapillary escape rate of albumin and plasma volume in essential hypertension. Circ Res 32: 643-651, 1973.

745. Patel DJ, Frankel BL, Horwitz D, Mott DE. A control procedure for studies of blood pressure feedback in hypertension. Cardiovas Med 3: 627 and 630, 1978.

746. Patterson GC, Shephard JT, Whelan RF. The resistance to blood flow in the upper and lower limb vessels in patients with coarctation of the aorta. Clin Sci 16: 627-632, 1957.

747. Patterson JL Jr, Goetz RH, Doyle JT, Warren JV, Gauer OH, Detweiler DK, Said SI, Hoernicke H, McGregor M, Keen EN, Smith MH Jr, Hardie EL, Reynolds M, Flatt WP, Waldo DR. Cardiorespiratory dynamics in the ox and giraffe, with comparative observations on man and other mammals. Ann NY Acad Sci 27: 393-412, 1965.

748. Peart WS. Hypertension and the kidney. II. Experimental basis of renal hypertension. Brit Med J 2: 1421-1429, 1959.

749. Pedersen AH. A method of producing experimental chronic hypertension in the rabbit. Arch Pathol 3: 912, 1927.

750. Pedersen EB, Christensen NJ. Catecholamines in plasma and urine in patients with essential hypertension determined by double-isotope derivation techniques. Acta Med Sci 198: 373-377, 1975.

751. Pederson EB, Kornerup HJ. Renal haemodynamics and plasma renin in patients with essential hypertension. Clin Sci Molec 50: 409-414, 1976.

752. Perhach JL, Ferguson HC, McKinney GR. Evaluation of antihypertensive agents in the stress-induced hypertensive rat. Life Sci 16: 1731-1736, 1975.

753. Pfeffer JM, Pfeffer MA, Fishbein MC, Frohlich ED. Cardiac function and morphology with aging in the spontaneously hypertensive rat. Amer J Physiol 237: H461-H468, 1979.

754. Pfeffer JM, Pfeffer MA, Frohlich ED. Validity of an indirect tail-cuff method for determining systolic arterial pressure in unanesthetized normotensive and spontaneously hypertensive rats. J Lab Clin Med 78: 957-962, 1971.

755. Pfeffer MA, Frohlich ED. Hemodynamic and myocardial function in young and old normotensive and spontaneously hypertensive rats. Circ Res 32(Suppl I): 28-35, 1973.

756. Pfeffer MA, Pfeffer JM, Weiss AK, Frohlich ED. Development of SHR hypertension and cardiac hypertrophy during prolonged beta blockade. Amer J Physiol 232: H639-H644, 1977.

757. Phelan EL. Cardiovascular reactivities in rats with spontaneous inherited hypertension and constricted renal arteries. Amer Heart J 71: 50-57, 1966.

758. Pickering GW. The peripheral resistance in persistent arterial hypertension. Clin Sci 2: 209-235, 1935.

759. Pickering GW. Role of the kidney in acute and chronic hypertension following renal artery constriction in the rabbit. Clin Sci 5: 229-247, 1945.

760. Pickering G. The inheritance of arterial pressure. pp 18-25 in _The Epidemiology of Hypertension_, eds J Stamler, R Stamler, TN Pullman. Grune and Stratton, New York, 1967.

761. Pickering G. _Hypertension : Causes, Consequences and Management_. Williams and Wilkens, Baltimore, 1970.

762. Pitcock JA, Brown PS, Brooks B, Clapp WL, Brosius WL, Muirhead EE. Renomedullary deficiency in partial nephrectomy-salt hypertension. Hypertension 2: 281-290, 1980.

763. Planz G, Planz R. Dopamine-beta-hydroxylase, adrenaline, noradrenaline and dopamine in the venous blood of adrenal gland of man: A comparison with levels in the periphery of the circulation. Experientia 35: 207-208, 1979.

764. Platt R. Heredity in hypertension. Lancet 1: 899-904, 1963.

765. Plotz CM, Knowlton AI, Ragan C. The natural history of Cushing's syndrome. Amer J Med 13: 597-614, 1952.

766. Pomeranz BH, Birtch AG, Barger AC. Neural control of intrarenal blood flow. Amer J Physiol 215: 1067-1081, 1968.

767. Port S, Cobb FR, Jones RH. Effects of propranolol on left ventricular function in normal men. Circulation 61: 358-366, 1980.

768. Postnov YV, Orlov SN, Shevchenko A, Adler AM. Altered sodium permeability, calcium binding and Na-K-ATPase activity in the red blood cell membrane in essential hypertension. Pflueger Arch 371: 263-269, 1977.

769. Prewitt RL, Dowell RF. Structural vascular adaptations during the developmental stages of hypertension in the spontaneously hypertensive rat. Bibl Anat 18: 169-173, 1979.

770. Prichard BNC, Gillam PMS. Use of propranolol (Inderal) in treatment of hypertension. Brit Med J 2: 725-727, 1964.

771. Prichard BNC, Gillam PMS. Treatment of hypertension with propranolol. Brit Med J 7-16, 1969.

772. Priddle WW. Observations on the management of hypertension. Canad Med Ass J 25: 5-8, 1931.

773. Prior IAM, Grimley-Evans JG, Harvey HPB, Davidson F, Lindsey M. Sodium intake and blood pressure in two Polynesian populations. New Eng J Med 279: 515-520, 1968.

774. Provoost AP, DeJong W. Differential development of renal, DOCA-salt, and spontaneous hypertension in the rat after neonatal sympathectomy. Clin Exp Hyperten 1: 177-189, 1978.

775. Pullan PT, Johnston WP, Korner PI. Plasma vasopressin in blood pressure homeostasis and in experimental renal hypertension. Amer J Physiol 239:

H81-H87, 1980.

776. Ragan C, Bordley J. The accuracy of clinical measurements of arterial blood pressure. Bull Johns Hopkins Hosp 69: 504-528, 1941.

777. Randall O, Esler M, Culp B, Julius S, Zweifler A. Determinants of baroreflex sensitivity in man. J Lab Clin Med 91: 514-519, 1978.

778. Rapp JP, Bergon L. Characteristics of pituitary colloid proteins and their correlation with blood pressure in the rat. Endocrinology 101: 93-103, 1977.

779. Rapp JP, Dahl LK. Mendelian inheritance of 18 and 11-beta steroid hydroxylase activities in the adrenals of rats genetically susceptible or resistant to hypertension. Endocrinology 90: 1435-1446, 1972.

780. Rapp JP, Dahl LK. Anatomical and protein electrophoretic observation on pituitary cleft colloid in rats genetically susceptible or resistant to salt hypertension. Lab Invest 30: 417-426, 1974.

781. Rapp JP, Knudsen KD, Iwai J, Dahl LK. Genetic control of blood pressure and corticosteroid production in rats. Circ Res 32(Suppl I): 139-149, 1973.

782. Rapp JP, McPartland RP, Sustarsic DL. Inheritance of blood pressure and pituitary colloid protein in Dahl rats. J Heredity 10: 169-174, 1979.

783. Rapp JP, Tan SY, Margolius HS. Plasma mineralocorticoids, plasma renin, and urinary kallikrein in salt-sensitive and salt-resistant rats. Endocr Res Comm 5: 35-41, 1978.

784. Redleaf PD, Tobian L. Sodium restriction and reserpine administration in experimental hypertension. Circ Res 6: 343-351, 1958.

785. Regoli D, Ganthier R. Site of action of angiotensin and the other vasoconstrictors on the kidney. Canad J Physiol Pharmacol 49: 608-612, 1971.

786. Regoli D, Hess R, Brunner H, Peters G, Gross F. Interrelationships of renin content in kidneys and

blood pressure in renal hypertensive rats. Arch Inter Pharmacodyn 140: 416-426, 1962.

787. Regoli D, Park WK, Rioux F. Pharmacology of angiotensin. Pharmacol Rev 26: 69-123, 1974.

788. Reid JL, Dargie HJ, Franklin SS, Fraser B. Plasma noradrenaline and renovascular hypertension in the rat. Clin Sci Molec Med 51: 439s-442s, 1976.

789. Reid JL, Zivin JA, Kopin IJ. Central and peripheral adrenergic mechanisms in the development of deoxycorticosterone-saline hypertension in rats. Circ Res 37: 569-579, 1975.

790. Reisin E, Abel R, Modan M, Silverberg DS, Eliahou HE, Modan B. Effect of weight loss without salt restriction on the reduction of blood pressure in overweight hypertensive patients. New Eng J Med 298: 1-6, 1978.

791. Reubi FC. Renal hyperemia induced in man by a new phthalazine derivative. Proc Soc Exp Biol Med 73: 102-103, 1950.

792. Reubi FC, Weidmann P, Hodler J, Cottier PT. Changes in renal function in essential hypertension. Amer J Med 64: 556-563, 1978.

793. Reybrouck T, Amery A, Billiet L. Hemodynamic response to graded exercise after chronic beta-adrenergic blockade. J Appl Physiol: Respirat Environ Exercise Physiol 42: 133-138, 1977.

794. Ribeiro AB, Krakoff LR. The adrenal component of renal hypertension. Circulation 54(Suppl II): 177, 1976.

795. Richardson TQ, Fermoso JD, Guyton AC. Increase in mean circulatory pressure in Goldblatt hypertension. Amer J Physiol 207: 751-752, 1964.

796. Riegger AJG, Lever AF, Millar JA, Morton JJ, Slack B. Correction of renal hypertension in the rat by prolonged infusion of angiotensin inhibitors. Lancet 2: 1317-1319, 1977.

797. Rippe B, Lundin S, Folkow B. Plasma volume, blood volume and transcapillary escape rate of albumin in

young spontaneously hypertensive rats as compared to normotensive controls. Clin Exp Hyperten 1: 39-50, 1978.

798. Robie NW, McNay JL. Comparative splanchnic blood flow effects of various vasodilator compounds. Circ Shock 4: 69-78, 1977.

799. Rocchini AP, Barger AC. Renovascular hypertension in sodium-depleted dogs: role of renin and carotid sinus reflex. Amer J Physiol 236: H101-H107, 1979.

800. Rocchini AP, Rosenthal A, Barger AC, Costaneda AR, Nadas AS. Pathogenesis of paradoxical hypertension after coarctation resection. Circulation 54: 382-387, 1976.

801. Rocha e Silva M Jr, Rosenberg M. The release of vasopressin in response to haemorrhage and its role in the mechanism of blood pressure regulation. J Physiol 202: 535-559, 1969.

802. Roizen MF, Weise V, Grobecker H, Kopin IJ. Plasma catecholamines and dopamine-beta-hydroxylase activity in spontaneously hypertensive rats. Life Sci 17: 283-288, 1975.

803. Romero JC, Kozak TJ, Hoobler SW. The effect of nephrectomy and of renomedullary extracts on the blood pressure of experimentally hypertensive rabbits. Proc Soc Exp Biol Med 140: 651-656, 1972.

804. Romero JC, Ott CE, Aguilo JJ, Torres VE, Strong CG. Role of prostaglandin in the reversal of one-kidney hypertension in the rat. Circ Res 37: 683-689, 1975.

805. Rosas R, Gomez A, Montague D, Gross M, Hoobler SW. Hemodynamic effects of renal transplants in hypertensive and control rats. Proc Soc Exp Biol Med 115: 4-8, 1964.

806. Rosen SM, Robinson PJA. Interdependence of exchangeable sodium and plasma renin concentration in determining blood pressure in patients treated by maintenance dialysis. Brit Med J 4: 139-143, 1973.

807. Rothe CF. A computer model of the cardiovascular system for effective learning. Physiologist 22:

29-33, 1979.

808. Rothlin E, Cerletti A, Emmenegger HE. Experimental psycho-neurogenic hypertension and its treatment with hydrogenated ergot alkaloids (Hydergine). Acta Med Scand Suppl 312: 27-35, 1956.

809. Rubin AA, Roth FE, Taylor RM, Rosenkilde H. Pharmacology of diazoxide, an antihypertensive, nondiuretic benzothiadiazine. J Pharmacol Exp Ther 136: 344-352, 1962.

810. Rubin B, Antonaccio MJ, Goldberg ME, Harris DN, Itkin AG, Horovitz ZP, Panasevich RE, Laffan RJ. Chronic antihypertensive effects of captopril (SQ 14225), an orally active angiotensin I converting enzyme inhibitor, in conscious two-kidney renal hypertensive rats. Europ J Pharmacol 51: 377-388, 1978.

811. Russek HI, Rath MM, Zohman BL, Miller I. Influence of age on blood pressure: Study of 5,331 white male subjects. Amer Heart J 32: 468-479, 1946.

812. Rytand DA. Pathogenesis of arterial hypertension in coarctation of the aorta. Proc Soc Exp Biol Med 38: 10-11, 1938.

813. Rytand DA. The renal factor in arterial hypertension with coarctation of the aorta. J Clin Invest 17: 391-399, 1938.

814. Safar ME, Chau NP, Weiss YA, London GM, Milliez PL. Control of cardiac output in essential hypertension. Amer J Cardiol 38: 332-336, 1976.

815. Safar ME, London GM, Levenson JA, Simon AC, Chau NP. Rapid dextran infusion in essential hypertension. Hypertension 1: 615-623, 1979.

816. Safar ME, London GM, Weiss YA, Milliez PL. Altered blood volume regulation in sustained essential hypertension: A hemodynamic study. Kid Inter 8: 42-47, 1975.

817. Safar ME, London GM, Weiss YA, Milliez PL. Overhydration and renin failure: a hemodynamic study. Clin Nephrol 5: 183-188, 1975.

818. Safar ME, Milliez P. Hemodynamic findings in human

arterial hypertension. Rev Europ Etudes Clin et Biol 17: 147-154, 1972.

819. Safar ME, Weiss YA, Levenson JA, London GM, Milliez PL. Hemodynamic study of 85 patients with borderline hypertension. Amer J Cardiol 31: 315-319, 1973.

820. Salgado HC, Krieger EM. Reversibility of baroreceptor adaptation in chronic hypertension. Clin Sci Molec Med 45(Suppl): 123s-126s, 1973.

821. Salgado MCO, Kreiger EM. Cardiac output in unrestrained conscious rats. Clin Exp Pharmacol Physiol 3(Suppl): 165-167, 1976.

822. Salzano JV, Gunning RV, Mastopaulo TN, Tuttle WW. Effect of weight loss on blood pressure. J Amer Diet Ass 34: 1309-1312, 1958.

823. Samanek M, Goetzova J, Fiserova J, Skovranek J. Differences in muscle blood flow in upper and lower extremities of patients after correction of coarctation of the aorta. Circulation 54: 377-381, 1976.

824. Samar RE, Coleman TG. Mean circulatory pressure and vascular compliances in the spontaneously hypertensive rat. Amer J Physiol 237: H584-H589, 1979.

825. Samar RE, Coleman TG. Effects of sodium restriction and antihypertensive therapy in spontaneously hypertensive rats. Fed Proc 39: 1193, 1980.

826. Sasaki N. High blood pressure and the salt intake of the Japanese. Jap Heart J 3: 313-324, 1962.

827. Satoh S, Zimmerman BG. Effect of (Sar-1, Ala-8) angiotensin II on renal vascular resistance. Amer J Physiol 229: 640-645, 1975.

828. Schachter J. Pain, fear and anger in hypertensives and normotensives: A psychophysiologic study. Psychosom Med 19: 17-29, 1957.

829. Schackow E, Dahl LK. Effects of chronic excess salt ingestion: lack of gross salt retention in salt-hypertension. Proc Soc Exp Biol Med 122: 952-957, 1966.

830. Schaechtelin G. Regoli D, Gross F. Bio-assay of circulating renin-like pressor material by isovolemic cross circulation. Amer J Physiol 205: 303-306, 1963.

831. Schalekamp MADH, Birkenhager WH. Renin levels in hypertension. New Eng J Med 286: 1319-1320, 1972.

832. Schalekamp MADH, Krauss XH, Kolsters G, Schalekamp MPA, Birkenhager WH. Renin suppression in hypertension in relation to body fluid volumes, patterns of sodium excretion and renal hemodynamics. Clin Sci Molec Med 45(Suppl): 283s-286s, 1973.

833. Schalekamp MADH, Schalekamp-Kuyken MPA, Birkenhager WH. Abnormal renal hemodynamics and renin suppression in hypertensive patients. Clin Sci 38: 101-110, 1970.

834. Scher AM. Carotid and aortic regulation of arterial blood pressure. Circulation 56: 521-528, 1977.

835. Schimert P, Kezdi P, Nishimura T. The effect of pituitary stalk-section on neurogenic and renal hypertension in the dog. Arch Inter Pharmacodyn 147: 236-254, 1964.

836. Schlager G. Spontaneous hypertension in laboratroy animals. A review of the genetic implications. J Hered 63: 35-38, 1972.

837. Schlager G. Selection for blood pressure levels in mice. Genetics 76: 537-549, 1974.

838. Schlierf G, Arab L, Schellenberg B, Oster P, Mordasini R, Schmidt-Gayk H, Vogel G. Salt and hypertension: data from the "Heidelberg Study". Amer J Clin Nutrit 33: 872-875, 1980.

839. Schmidlin J, Anner G, Billeter JR, Wettstein A. Uber synthesen in der Aldosteron-Reihe I. Totalsynthese des racemischen Aldosterons. Experientia 11: 365-368, 1955.

840. Schomig A, Dietz R, Rascher W. Regulation of the intravascular volume and of the total peripheral resistance in spontaneous hypertensive rats. Bibl Anat 18: 177-179, 1979.

841. Schomig A, Szokol M, Dietz R, Luth B, Gross F. Fluid and salt intake during the development of renal hypertension in rats. Clin Exp Pharmacol Physiol 7: 169-182, 1980.

842. Schwartz WB. The effect of sulfanilamide on salt and water excretion in congestive heart failure. New Eng J Med 240: 173-177, 1949.

843. Schwietzer G, Gertz KH. Changes of hemodynamics and glomerular ultrafiltration in renal hypertension of rats. Kid Inter 15: 134-143, 1979.

844. Scoggins BA, Butkus A, Coghlan JP, Denton DA, Fan JSK, Humphrey TJ, Whitworth JA. Adrenocorticotropic hormone-induced hypertension in sheep. Circ Res 43(Suppl I): 76-81, 1978.

845. Scoggins BA, Coghlan JP, Cran EJ, Denton DA, Fan SK, McDougall JG, Oddie CJ, Robinson PM, Shulkes AA. Experimental studies on the mechanism of adrenocorticotrophic hormone induced hypertension in sheep. Clin Sci 45: 269s-271s, 1973.

846. Scoggins BA, Coghlan JP, Denton DA, Fan JSK, McDougall JG, Oddie CJ, Shulkes AA. Metabolic effects of ACTH in the sheep. Amer J Physiol 226: 198-205, 1974.

847. Scott HW, Bahnson HT. Evidence for a renal factor in the hypertension of experimental coarctation of the aorta. Surgery 30: 206-217, 1951.

848. Scott HW, Collins HA, Langa AM, Olsen NS. Additional observations concerning the physiology of the hypertension associated with experimental coarctation of the aorta. Surgery 36: 445-459, 1954.

849. Scriabine A. Beta-adrenoceptor blocking drugs in hypertension. Ann Rev Pharmacol Toxicol 19: 269-284, 1979.

850. Seebes AM, Arranz CT. Body fluid changes in hypertensive rats. Their modifications by saline load. Nephron 24: 241-245, 1979.

851. Selkurt EE. Effect of pulse pressure and mean arterial pressure modification on renal hemodynamics and electrolyte and water excretion. Circulation 4:

541-551, 1951.

852. Selkurt EE, Abel FL, Edwards JL, Yum MN. Renal function in dogs with hypertension induced by immunologic nephritis. Proc Soc Exp Med Biol 144: 295-303, 1973.

853. Sen S, Smeby RR, Bumpus FM. Renin in rats with spontaneous hypertension. Circ Res 31: 876-880, 1972.

854. Sever PS, Osikowska B, Birch M, Tunbridge RDG. Plasma noradrenaline in essential hypertension. Lancet 1: 1078-1081, 1977.

855. Shapiro AP. An experimental study of comparative responses of blood pressure to different noxious stimuli. J Chronic Dis 13: 293-311, 1961.

856. Shapiro AP, Braude AI, Siemienski J. Hematogenous pyelonephritis in rats. IV. Relationship and sequelae of chronic pyelonephrites. J Clin Invest 38: 1228-1240, 1959.

857. Shapiro AP, Schwartz GE, Ferguson DCE, Redmond DP, Weiss SM. Behavioral methods in the treatment of hypertension. I. Review of their clinical status. Ann Inter Med 86: 626-636, 1977.

858. Sheps DS, Schrumpf JD, Aronson AL, Wolfson S, Cohen LS. Propranolol and oxygen-hemoglobin equilibrium. Circulation 50: 864-865, 1974.

859. Shipley RE, Study RS. Changes in renal blood flow, extraction of inulin, glomerular filtration rate, tissue pressure and urine flow with acute alterations of renal artery pressure. Amer J Physiol 167: 676-688, 1951.

860. Siegel MB, Levinsky NG. Collateral circulation after renal artery occlusion in the rat. Circ Res 41: 227-231, 1977.

861. Simon AC, Safar ME, Levenson JA, London GM, Levy BI, Chau NP. An evaluation of large arteries compliance in man. Amer J Phsiol 237: H550-H554, 1979.

862. Simon AC, Safar ME, Weiss YA, London GM, Milliez PL. Baroreflex sensitivity and cardiopulmonary blood

volume in normotensive and hypertensive patients. Brit Heart J 39: 799-805, 1977.

863. Simon G. Altered venous function in hypertensive rats. Circ Res 38: 412-418, 1976.

864. Simon G, Franciosa JA, Cohn JN. Decreased venous distensibility in essential hypertension: Lack of systemic hemodynamic correlates. Angiology 30: 147-159, 1979.

865. Simon G, Pamnani MB, Dunkel JF, Overbeck HW. Mesenteric hemodynamics in early experimental renal hypertension in dogs. Circ Res 36: 791-798, 1975.

866. Simpson FO, Phelan EL, Lee DR, Jones DR, Butt TJ, Ledingham JM, Bolli P. Body fluids, sodium and renal blood flow distribution in the New Zealand genetically hypertensive rat. pp 137-143 in The Kidney in Arterial Hypertension, eds G Bianchi, G Bazzato. Bunge Scientific Publishers, Utrecht, 1979.

867. Simpson SA, Tait JF, Wettstein A, Neher R, Von Euw J, Reichstein T. Isolieurung eines neun Kristavlisierten hormons aus nebennieren mit besonders hoher wirksamkeit auf den mineralstoffwechsel. Experientia 9: 333-335, 1953.

868. Simpson SA, Tait JR, Wettstein A, Neher R, Von Euw J, Schindler O, Reichstein T. Konstitution des aldosterons des neuen mineralocorticoids. Experientia 10: 132-133, 1954.

869. Sims EAH, Phinney SD, Vaswani A. The management of hypertension associated with obesity. Inter J Obes 2: 215-223, 1978.

870. Singer B, Losito C, Salmon S. Aldosterone and corticosterone secretion rates in rats with experimental renal hypertension. Acta Endocrinol 44: 505-518, 1963.

871. Sinnett PF, Whyte NM. Epidemiological studies in a total highland population. Tukisenta, New Guinea. Cardiovascular disease and relevant clinical, electrocardiographic, radiological and biochemical findings. J Chronic Dis 26: 265-290, 1973.

872. Sivertsson R, Hansson E, Eriksson B. Hemodynamic

signs indicating structural vascular changes of hypertensive type after surgery for aortic coarctation. Acta Med Scand S625: 116-121, 1979.

873. Sivertsson R, Hansson L. Effects of blood pressure reduction on the structural vascular abnormality in skin and muscle vascular beds in human essential hypertension. Clin Sci Molec Med 51(Suppl III): 77-79, 1976.

874. Sivertsson R, Olander R. Aspects of the nature of the increased vascular resistance and increased "reactivity" to noradrenalin in hypertensive subjects. Life Sci 7: 1291-1297, 1968.

875. Sivertsson R, Sannerstedt R, Lundgren Y. Evidence for peripheral vascular involvement in mild elevation of blood pressure in man. Clin Sci Molec Med 51(Suppl III): 65-68, 1976.

876. Skeggs LT, Marsh WH, Kahn JR, Shumway NP. Amino acid composition and electrophoretic properties of hypertensin I. J Exp Med 102: 435-440, 1955.

877. Sleight P. Neural control of the cardiovascular system. Mod Trends Cardiol 3: 1-43, 1974.

878. Slick GL, Aguilera AJ, Zambraski EJ, DiBona GF, Kaloyanides GJ. Renal neuroadrenergic transmission. Amer J Physiol 229: 60-65, 1975.

879. Smirk FH, Hall WH. Inheritied hypertension in rats. Nature 182: 727-728, 1958.

880. Smith MJ Jr, Cowley AW Jr, Guyton AC, Manning RD Jr. Acute and chronic effects of vasopressin on blood pressure, electrolytes, and fluid volumes. Amer J Physiol 237: F232-F240, 1979.

881. Smith TL, Hutchins PM. Central hemodynamics in the development stage of spontaneous hypertension in the unanesthetized rat. Hypertension 1: 508-517, 1979.

882. Smithwick RH, Thompson JE. Splanchnicectomy for essential hypertension. JAMA 152: 1501-1504, 1953.

883. Smyth HS, Sleight P, Pickering GW. Reflex regulation of arterial pressure during sleep in man. Circ Res 24: 109-121, 1969.

884. Snyder DW, Doba N, Reis DJ. Regional distribution of blood flow during arterial hypertension produced by lesions of the nucleus tractus solitarii in rats. Circ Res 42: 87-91, 1978.

885. Snyder DW, Nathan MA, Reis DJ. Chronic lability of arterial pressure produced by selective destruction of the catecholamine innervation of the nucleus tractus solitarii in the rat. Circ Res 43: 662-671, 1978.

886. Sobin SS. Accuracy of indirect determinations of blood pressure in the rat. Amer J Physiol 146: 179-186, 1946.

887. Solez K, Jaenike JR, Richter GW. Polyuria, hypertension and altered renal function in experimental microembolic renal disease. Lab Invest 27: 243-253, 1972.

888. Sparks JC, Susic D. The effects of propranolol on plasma renin activity and renal renin concentration in rats on normal and sodium deficient diets. Pharmacol Res Comm 9: 479-487, 1977.

889. Sparks RF, Arkey A, Boulter PR, Saudek CD, O'Brian JT. Renin, aldosterone and glucagon in the natriuresis of fasting. New Eng J Med 292: 1335-1340, 1975.

890. Stamler R, Stamler J, Reidlinger WF, Algera G, Roberts RH. Weight and blood pressure. Findings in hypertension screening of 1 million Americans. JAMA 240: 1607-1610, 1978.

891. Steele JM. Comparison of simultaneous indirect (auscultatory) and direct (intra-arterial) measurements of arterial pressure in man. J Mount Sinai Hosp NY 8: 1042-1050, 1941.

892. Steiger M, Reichstein T. Desoxy-cortico-steron (21-Oxy-progesteron) aus Delta 5-3-Oxy-atio-choleusaure. Helv Chim Acta 20: 1164-1179, 1937.

893. Stephens GA, Davis JO, Freeman RH , DeForrest JM, Early PM. Hemodynamic, fluid, and electrolyte changes in sodium-depleted, one-kidney, renal hypertensive dogs. Circ Res 44: 316-321, 1979.

894. Steptoe A. Psychological methods in treatment of hypertension: a review. Brit Heart J 39: 587-593, 1977.

895. Stewart JM, Ferreira SH, Greene LJ. Bradykinin potentiating peptide PCA-Lys-Trp-Ala-Pro. An inhibitor of the pulmonary inactivation of bradykinin and conversion of angiotensin I to II. Biochem Pharmacol 20: 1557-1567, 1971.

896. Stubberfield J, Sutherland HD. The results of surgical treatment of coarctation of the thoracic aorta. Aust New Zeal J Surg 47: 36-40, 1977.

897. Sturkie PD, Weiss HS, Ringer RK, Sheahan MM. Heritability of blood pressure in chickens. Poult Sci 38: 333-337, 1959.

898. Sullivan JM, Adams DF, Hollenberg NK. Beta-Adrenergic blockade in essential hypertension. Circ Res 39: 532-536, 1976.

899. Susic D, Kentera D. Role of the renal medulla in the resistance of rats to salt hypertension. Pfluegers Arch 384: 283-285, 1980.

900. Susic D, Sparks JC, Kentera D. Suppressed antihypertensive function of the renal medulla in rats with spontaneous hypertension. Pflueger Arch 368: 173-175, 1977.

901. Susic D, Sparks JC, Machado EA, Kentera D. The mechanism of renomedullary antihypertensive action: hemodynamic studies in hydronephrotic rats with one-kidney renal clip hypertension. Clin Sci Molec Med 54: 361-367, 1978.

902. Swales JD, Tange JD. The influence of acute sodium depletion on experimental hypertension in the rat. J Lab Clin Med 78: 369-379, 1971.

903. Swales JD, Thurston H, Queiroz FP, Medina A. δdium balance during the development of experimental hypertension. J Lab Clin Med 80: 539-547, 1972.

904. Swales JD, Thurston H, Queiroz FP, Medina A, Holland J. Dual mechanism for experimental hypertension. Lancet 2: 1181-1183, 1971.

905. Swartz SL, Williams GH, Hollenberg NK, Moore TJ, Dluhy RG. Converting enzyme inhibition in essential hypertension: The hypotensive response does not reflect only reduced angiotensin II formation. Hypertension 1: 106-111, 1979.

906. Tadepalli AS, Walsh GM, Tobia AJ. Normal cardiac output in the conscious young spontaneously hypertensive rat: evidence for higher oxygen utilization. Life Sci 15: 1103-1114, 1975.

907. Takeda K, Bunag RD. Augumented sympathetic nerve activity and pressor responsiveness in DOCA hypertensive rats. Hypertension 2: 97-101, 1980.

908. Takeda K, Bunag RD. Chronic propranolol treatment inhibits sympathetic nerve activity and keeps blood pressure from rising in spontaneously hypertensive rats. Hypertension 2: 228-235, 1980.

909. Takeshita A, Mark AL. Neurogenic contribution to hind quarters vasoconstriction during high sodium intake in Dahl strain of genetically hypertensive rat. Circ Res 43(Suppl I): 86-91, 1978.

910. Takeshita A, Mark AL. Decreased venous distensibility in borderline hypertension. Hypertension 1: 202-206, 1979.

911. Takeshita A, Mark AL. Decreased vasodilator capacity of forearm resistance vessels in borderline hypertension. Hypertension 2: 610-616, 1980.

912. Takeshita A, Mark AL, Brody MJ. Prevention of salt-induced hypertension in the Dahl strain by 6-hydroxydopamine. Amer J Physiol 236: H48-H52, 1979.

913. Takeshita A, Tanaka S, Kuroiwa A, Nakamura M. Reduced baroreceptor sensitivity in borderline hypertension. Circulation 51: 738-742, 1975.

914. Talman WT, Snyder D, Reis DJ. Chronic lability of arterial pressure produced by destruction of A2 catecholaminergic neurons in rat brainstem. Circ Res 46: 842-853, 1980.

915. Tanaka T, Seki A, Fujii J, Kurihara H, Ikeda M. Norepinephrine turnover in two types of experimental

renovascular hypertension of the rabbit. Jap Circ J 41: 881-882, 1977.

916. Tarazi RC, Dustan HP, Bravo EL. Hemodynamic effects of propranolol in hypertension: a review. Postgrad Med J 52(Suppl 4): 92-100, 1976.

917. Tarazi RC, Dustan HP, Frohlich ED. Long-term thiazide therapy in essential hypertension: Evidence for persistent alteration in plasma volume and renin activity. Circulation 61: 709-717, 1970.

918. Tarazi RC, Frohlich ED, Dustan HP. Plasma volume in men with essential hypertension. New Eng J Med 278: 762-765, 1968.

919. Taylor AA, Pool JL, Lake CR, Ziegler MG, Rosen RA, Rollins DE, Mitchell JR. Plasma norepinephrine concentrations: no differences among normal volunteers and low, high or normal renin hypertensive patients. Life Sci 22: 1499-1510, 1978.

920. Ten Berg RGM, Leenen FHH, de Jong W. Plasma renin activity and sodium, potassium and water excretion during reversal of hypertension in the one-clip, two-kidney hypertensive rat. Clin Sci 57: 47-52, 1979.

921. Terris JM, Berecek KH, Cohen EL, Stanley JC, Whitehouse WM Jr, Bohr DF. Deoxycorticosterone hypertension in the pig. Clin Sci Molec Med 51(Suppl III): 303s-305s, 1976.

922. Terry AH Jr. Obesity and hypertension JAMA 81: 1283-1284, 1923.

923. Thal AP, Grage TB, Vernier RL. Function of the contralateral kidney in renal hypertension due to renal artery stenosis. Circulation 27: 36-43, 1963.

924. Thompson JMA, Dickinson CJ. The relation between the excretion of sodium and water and the perfusion pressure in the isolated, blood perfused, rabbit kidney, with special reference to changes occuring in clip-hypertension. Clin Sci Molec Med 50: 223-236, 1976.

925. Thurau K, Deetzen P. Die Diurese bei arteriellen Drucksteigerungen. Pflueger Arch 294: 567-580,

1962.

926. Thurston H, Bing RF, Marks ES, Swales JD. Response of chronic renovascular hypertension to surgical correction or prolonged blockade of the renin-angiotensin system by two inhibitors in the rat. Clin Sci 58: 15-20, 1980.

927. Thurston H, Bing RF, Swales JD. Reversal of two-kidney , one-clip renovascular hypertension in the rat. Hypertension 2: 256-265, 1980.

928. Thurston H, Swales JD. Influence of sodium restriction upon two models of renal hypertension. Clin Sci Molec Med 51: 275-279, 1976.

929. Thurston H, Swales JD. Converting enzyme inhibitor and saralasin infusion in rats. Circ Res 42: 588-592, 1978.

930. Tibblin G, Bergentz SE, Bjure J, Wilhelmsen L. Hematocrit, plasma protein, plasma volume, and viscosity in early hypertensive disease. Amer Heart J 72: 165-176, 1966.

931. Tidball CS. A digital computer simulation of cardiovascular and renal physiology. Physiologist 22: 37-43, 1979.

932. Tigerstedt R, Bergman PG. Niere und Kreislauf. Scand Arch Physiol 8: 223-271, 1898.

933. Tobian L. Why do thiazide diuretics lower blood pressure in hypertension? Ann Rev Pharmacol 7: 399-408, 1967.

934. Tobian L, Coffee K, McCrea P. Contrasting exchangeable sodium in rats with different types of Goldblatt hypertension. Amer J Physiol 217: 458-460, 1969.

935. Tobian L, Lange J, Azar S, Iwai J, Koop D, Coffee K, Johnson MA. Reduction of natriuretic capacity and renin release in isolated, blood perfused kidneys of Dahl hypertension-prone rats. Circ Res 43(Suppl I): 92-98, 1978.

936. Tobian L, Lange J, Iwai J, Hiller K, Johnson MA, Goossens P. Prevention with thiazide of NaCl-induced

hypertension in Dahl "S" rats. Hypertension 1: 316-323, 1979.

937. Tobian L, Thompson J, Twedt R, Janecek J. The granulation of juxtaglomerular cells in renal hypertension, deoxycorticosterone and postdeoxcorticosterone hypertension, adrenal regeneration hypertension and adrenal insufficiency. Clin Invest 37: 660-671, 1958.

938. Trippodo NC, Walsh GM, Ferrone RA, Dugan RC. Fluid partition and cardiac output in volume-depleted Goldblatt hypertensive rats. Amer J Physiol 237: H18-H24, 1979.

939. Trippodo NC, Walsh GM, Frohlich ED. Fluid volumes during onset of spontaneous hypertension in rats. Amer J Physiol 235: H52-H58, 1978.

940. Truett J, Cornfield J, Kannel WB. A multivariate analysis of the risk of coronary heart disease in Framingham. J Chronic Dis 20: 511-524, 1967.

941. Tseng WP. Blood pressure and hypertension in an agricultural and a fishing population in Taiwan. Amer J Epidem 86: 513-525, 1967.

942. Tuck ML, Williams GH, Dluhy RG, Greenfield M, Moore TJ. A delayed suppression of the renin-aldosterone axis folloeing saline infusion in human hypertension. Circ Res 39: 711-717, 1976.

943. Ulrych M. Plasma volume decrease and elevated Evans Blue disappearance rate in essential hypertension. Clin Sci Molec Med 45: 173-181, 1973.

944. Ulrych M, Frohlich ED, Dustan HP, Page IH. Immediate hemodynamic effects of beta-adrenergic blockade with propranolol in normotensive and hypertensive man. Circulation 37: 411-416, 1968.

945. Ulrych M, Hofman J, Hejl Z. Cardiac and renal hyperresponsiveness to acute plasma volume expansion in hypertension. Amer Heart J 68: 193-203, 1964.

946. Valtin H. Hereditary hypothalamic diabetes insipidus in rats (Brattleboro strain). Amer J Med 42: 814-827, 1967.

947. Valtin H, Schroeder HA, Benirschke K, Sokol HW. Familial hypothalamic diabetes insipidus in rats. Nature 196: 1109-1110, 1962.

948. van Ameringen MR, de Champlain J, Imbeault S. Participation of central noradrenergic neurons in experimental hypertension. Canad J Physiol Pharmacol 55: 1246-1251, 1977.

949. van Brummelen P, Man in't Veld AJ, Schalekamp MADH. Hemodynamic changes during long-term thiazide treatment of essential hypertension in responders and nonresponders. Clin Pharmacol Ther 27: 328-336, 1980.

950. van Brummelen P, Schalekamp MADH. Body fluid volumes and the response of renin and aldosterone to short- and long-term thiazide therapy of hypertension. Acta Med Scand 207: 259-264, 1980.

951. van Brummelen P, Woerlee M, Schalekamp MADH. Long-term versus short-term effects of hydrochlorothiazide on renal hemodynamics in essential hypertension. Clin Sci 56: 463-469, 1979.

952. Van Citters RL, Kemper WS, Franklin DL. Blood pressure responses of wild giraffes studied by radio telemetry. Science 152: 384-386, 1966.

953. Vander AJ, Henry JP, Stephens PM, Kay LL, Mouw DR. Plasma renin activity in psychosocial hypertension of CBA mice. Circ Res 42: 496-502, 1978.

954. Vandermolen R, Brewer G, Honeyman MS, Morrison J, Hoobler SW. A study of hypertension in twins. Amer Heart J 79: 454-457, 1970.

955. Van Way CW, Michelabeis AM, Anderson WJ, Manlove A, Oates JA. Studies of plasma renin activity in coarctation of the aorta. Ann Surg 183: 229-238, 1976.

956. Vapaatalo H, Hackman R, Anttila P, Vainronpaa V, Neuvonen. Effects of 6-hydroxydopamine on spontaneously hypertensive rats. Naunyn-Schmiedeberg Arch Pharmacol 284: 1-13, 1974.

957. Vaughan ED Jr, Carey RM, Peach MJ, Ackerly JA, Ayers CR. The renin response to diuretic therapy: A

limitation of antihypertensive potential. Circ Res 42: 376-381, 1978.

958. Verney EB. Polyuria in chronic nephritis. Lancet 1: 751-756, 1929.

959. Vertes C, Cangiano JL, Berman LB, Gould A. Hypertension in end-stage renal disease. New Eng J Med 280: 978-981, 1969.

960. Veterans Administration Cooperative Study Group on Antihypertensive Agents. Effects of treatment on morbidity in hypertension. Results in patients with diastolic blood pressures averaging 115 through 129 mmHg. JAMA 202: 1028-1034, 1957.

961. Veterans Administration Cooperative Study Group in Antihypertensive Agents. Effects of treatment on morbidity in hypertension. II. Results in patients with diastolic blood pressure averaging 90-114 mmHg. JAMA 213: 1143-1152, 1970.

962. Veterans Administration Cooperative Study Group on Antihypertensive Agents. Effects of treatment on morbidity in hypertension. III. Influence of age, diastolic pressure and prior cardiovascular disease; further analysis of side effects. Circulation 45: 991-1004, 1972.

963. Villamil MF, Matloff J. Changes in vascular ionic content and distribution across aortic coarctation in the dog. Amer J Physiol 228: 1087-1093, 1975.

964. Vlachakis ND. Blood pressure variability and plasma catecholamines in man. Effect of propranolol therapy. Biochem Med 21: 253-261, 1979.

965. Vogel JA. Salt-induced hypertension in the dog. Amer J Physiol 210: 186-190, 1966.

966. Waeber B, Brunner HR, Brunner DB, Curtet AL, Turini GA, Gavras H. Discrepancy between antihypertensive effect and angiotensin converting enzyme inhibition by captopril. Hypertension 2: 236-242, 1980.

967. Wakerlin WE. From Bright toward light : The story of hypertension research. Circ Res 11: 131-136, 1962.

968. Wakim KG, Slaughter O, Clagett OT. Studies on the blood flow in the extremities in cases of coarctation of the aorta: Determinations before and after excision of the coarctate region. Mayo Clin, Proc Staff Meet 23: 347-351, 1948.

969. Wallin BG, Delius W, Hagbarth K. Comparison of sympathetic nerve activity in normotensive and hypertensive subjects. Circ Res 33: 9-21, 1973.

970. Wallin BG, Sundlof G. A quantitative study of muscle nerve sympathetic activity in resting normotensive and hypertensive subjects. Hypertension 1: 67-77, 1979.

971. Walsh JA, Hyman C, Maronde RF. Venous distensibility in essential hypertension. Cardiol Res 3: 338-349, 1969.

972. Warren S, Chute RN. Pheochromocytoma. Cancer 29: 327-331, 1972.

973. Watkin DM, Froeb HF, Hatch FT, Gutman AB. Effects of diet in hypertension. Amer J Med 9: 441-493, 1950.

974. Watkins BE, Davis JO, Freeman RH, Stephens GA. Production of renovascular hypertension in adrenalectomized dogs. Physiologist 19: 405, 1976.

975. Watkins BE, Davis JO, Freeman RH, Stephens GA, DeForrest JM. Effects of the oral converting enzyme inhibitor (SQ 14225) on one-kidney hypertension in the dog. Proc Soc Exp Biol Med 157: 245-249, 1978.

976. Watkins BE, Davis JO, Hanson RC, Lohmeier TE, Freeman RH. Incidence and pathophysiological changes in chronic two-kidney hypertension in the dog. Amer J Physiol 231: 954-960, 1976.

977. Watson RDS, Stallard TJ, Littler WA. Effects of beta-adrenoceptor antagonists on sino-aortic baroreflex sensitivity and blood pressure in hypertensive man. Clin Sci 57: 241-247, 1979.

978. Waugh WH. Angiotensin II: Local renal effects of physiological increments in concentration. Canad J Physiol Pharmacol 50: 711-716, 1972.

979. Weidmann P, Beretta-Piccoli C, Ziegler WH, Keusch G,

Gluck Z, Reubi FC. Age versus urinary sodium for judging renin, aldosterone, and catecholamine levels: Studies in normal subjects and patients with essential hypertension. Kid Inter 14: 619-628, 1978.

980. Weidmann P, Maxwell MH, Lupu AN, Lewin AJ, Massry SG. Plasma renin activity and blood pressure in terminal renal failure. New Eng J Med 285: 757-762, 1971.

981. Weiss E. Psychosomatic aspects of hypertension. JAMA 120: 1081-1086, 1942.

982. Weiss L, Hallback M. Time course and extent of structural vascular adaptation to regional hypotension in adult spontaneously hypertensive rats. Acta Physiol Scand 91: 365-373, 1974.

983. Wen S-F, Wong NLM, Evanson RL, Lockhart EA, Dirks JH. Micropuncture studies of sodium transport in the remnant kidney of the dog. J Clin Invest 52: 386-397, 1973.

984. Whyte H. Behind the adipose curtain. Amer J Cardiol 15: 66-80, 1965.

985. Widimsky J, Fejfarova MH, Fejfar Z. Changes of cardiac output in hypertensive disease. Cardiologia 31: 381-389, 1957.

986. Wilburn RL, Blaufuss A, Bennett CM. Long-term treatment for severe hypertension with minoxidil, propranolol and furosemide. Circulation 52: 706-713, 1975.

987. Williams GH, Hollenberg NK. Accentuated vascular and endocrine response to SQ 20881 in hypertension. New Eng J Med 297: 184-188, 1977.

988. Williams JB, Harrison TR, Grollman A. A simple method for determining the systolic blood pressure in the unanesthetized rat. J Clin Invest 18: 373-376, 1939.

989. Wilson C, Byrom FB. Renal changes in malignant hypertension. Lancet 1: 136-139, 1939.

990. Wilson C, Byrom FB. Vicious cycle in chronic Bright's disease: Experimental evidence from the

hypertensive rat. Quart J Med 10: 65-93, 1941.

991. Winer BM. The antihypertensive actions of benzothiadiazines. Circulation 23: 211-218, 1961.

992. Winkelstein W Jr, Kantor S, Ibrahim M, Sackett DL. Familial aggregation of blood pressure. JAMA 195: 160-162, 1966.

993. Winternitz S, Katholi R, Oparil S. The contribution of enhanced renal sympathetic tone to the development of hypertension in the spontaneously hypertensive rat. Clin Res 27: 783A, 1979.

994. Wolf HJ, von Bonsdorff B. Blutige Messung der absoluten Sphygmogramms beim Menschen. Z Ges Exper Med 79: 569-577, 1931.

995. Wolf S, Pfeiffer JB, Ripley HS, Winter OS, Wolff HG. Hypertension as a reaction pattern to stress: Summary of experimental data on variations in blood pressure and renal blood flow. Ann Intern Med 29: 1056-1076, 1948.

996. Wright GL, Knecht E, Badger D, Samueloff S, Toraason M, Dukes-Dobos F. Oxygen consumption in the spontaneously hypertensive rat. Proc Soc Exp Biol Med 159: 449-452, 1978.

997. Wyatt RJ, Murphy DL, Belmaker R, Cohen S, Donelly CH, Pollin W. Reduced monoamine oxidase activity in platelets: a possible genetic marker for vulnerability to schizophrenia. Science 179: 916-918, 1973.

998. Yamamoto J, Trippodo NC, Ishise S, Frohlich ED. Altered pressure/volume relationship in one-kidney Goldblatt hypertensive rats. Fed Proc 38: 1258, 1979.

999. Yamori Y, Yamabe H, de Jong W, Lovenberg W, Sjoerdsma A. Effect of tissue norepinephrine depletion by 6-hydroxydopamine on blood pressure in spontaneously hypertensive rats. Europ J Pharmacol 17: 135-140, 1972.

1000. Ylitalo P, Gross F. Hemodynamic changes during the development of sodium- induced hypertension in subtotally nephrectomized rats. Acta Physiol Scand

106: 447-455, 1979.

1001. Young DB, Murray RH, Bengis RG, Markov AK. Experimental angiotensin II hypertension. Amer J Physiol 239: H391-H398, 1980.

1002. Young DF, Cholvin NR, Roth AC. Pressure drop across artificially induced stenosis in the femoral arteries of dogs. Circ Res 36: 735-743, 1975.

1003. Young DF, Tsai FY. Flow characteristics in models of arterial stenosis I. Steady flow. J Biomech 6: 395-410, 1973.

1004. Young DF, Tsai FY. Flow characteristics in models of arterial stenosis: II. Unsteady flow. J Biomech 6: 547-559, 1973.

1005. Young JB, Landsberg L. Suppression of sympathetic nervous system during fasting. Science 196: 1473-1475, 1977.

1006. Young JB, Mullen D, Landsberg L. Caloric restriction lowers blood pressure in the spontaneously hypertensive rat. Metabolism 27: 1711-1714, 1978.

1007. Yu R, Dickinson CJ. Neurogenic effects of angiotensin. Lancet 2: 1276-1277, 1965.

1008. Yu R, Dickinson CJ. The progressive pressor response to angiotensin in the rabbit. The role of the sympathetic nervous system. Arch Intern Pharmacodyn 191: 24-36, 1971.

1009. Zandberg P, Palkovits M, de Jong W. Effects of various lesions in the nucleus tractus solitarii of the rat on blood pressure, heart rate and cardiovascular reflex responses. Clin Exp Hyperten 1: 355-379, 1978.

1010. Zimmerman BG. Involvement of angiotensin-mediated renal vasoconstriction in renal hypertension. Life Sci 13: 507-515, 1973.

1011. Zinner SH, Levy PS, Kass EH. Familial aggregation of blood pressure in childhood. New Eng J Med 284: 401-404, 1971.

1012. Zweig SM, Rapoport A, Wilson DR, Ranking GN, Husdan H. The effects of chronic unilateral renal artery constriction on blood pressure, separate renal function, and the development of collateral circulation in the dog. Canad J Physiol Pharmacol 50: 1170-1180, 1972.

1013. Zweig SM, Rapoport A, Wilson DR, Ranking GN, Husdan H. Differential renal effects of angiotensin after unilateral renal artery constriction. J Appl Physiol 32: 859-863, 1972.

INDEX